Homeopathy in Veterinary Medicine

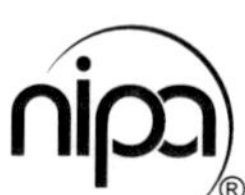

NIPA® GENX ELECTRONIC RESOURCES & SOLUTIONS P. LTD.
New Delhi-110 034

About the Author

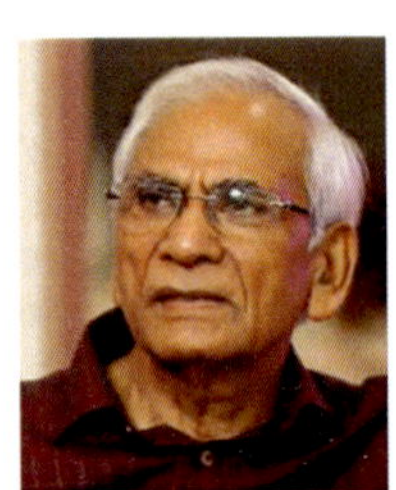

Prof. (Dr.) J.P. Varshney, a renowned veterinarian with a unique blend of academic, research and clinical experience of more than 58 years, is still busy in his clinical pursuits at Nandini Veterinary Hospital, Surat (Gujarat). Though trained in modern veterinary medicine, his research work on "Evaluation of homeopathic drugs in the management of various animal diseases" at premier Indian Veterinary Research Institute, not only sensitized veterinarians to Homeopathy in Veterinary Mdicine but also led to submission of few post graduate theses; publication of research papers in reputed journals (Homeopathy, Homoeopathic Links. International Journal of Classical Homeopathy, American Journal of Homeopathic Medicine, Homeopathy 4 Every One, Journal of Case Studies in Homeopathy, Indian Veterinary Journal, Indian Journal of Veterinary Medicine): a book on the "Research Findings -Homeopathic Bio efficacy and Management of Animal Health" : and many scientific and lead presentations in national and international conferences including World Homeopathic Summit-2015, Asian conference-2011, Liga-2010 and 2011, All India Homeopathic Conference 2014,National workshop on Alternate Medicine, Nagpur-2005, International Homeopathic Conferences (St. Petersburg, Canada, New Delhi), and many more. He has recently been honored at "New Frontiers in Homeopathy, a national conference - 3rd HOMEOPATHY VIJNANA SAMMELAN, Ahmedabad - 2023. Presently he has been nominated as a member Special Committee for Fundamental Research in Homoeopathy at Central Council for Research in Homeopathy, New Delhi. He has been bestowed with as many as 37 awards and honors including best teacher award, gold medals, and life time achievement awards. Besides publications in national and international journals of repute, he has eight books in the specialty of Veterinary Medicine at his credit.

Homeopathy in Veterinary Medicine

J.P. Varshney

B.V.Sc. and A.H.; M.V.Sc. (Veterinary Medicine)
Ph.D. (Veterinary Medicine)
Ex. Principal Scientist (Veterinary Medicine, IVRI, Izatnagar)
Senior Consultant (Veterinary Medicine)
Nandini Veterinary Hospital
Ghod-Dod Road, Surat-395001, Gujarat, India

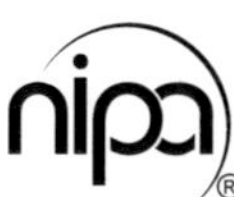

NIPA® GENX ELECTRONIC RESOURCES & SOLUTIONS P. LTD.

New Delhi-110 034

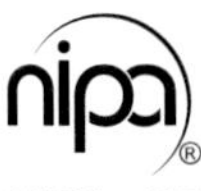

NIPA® GENX ELECTRONIC RESOURCES & SOLUTIONS P. LTD.

101,103, Vikas Surya Plaza, CU Block
L.S.C. Market, Pitam Pura, New Delhi-110 034
Ph : +91-11-43860225, Mob.: +91 9717133558, 9540816132
E-mail: newindiapublishingagency@gmail.com
Website: www.nipaersources.com

Print ISBN: 978-93-58879-15-5
ebook ISBN: 978-93-58879-58-2

Composed and Designed by NIPA®.

Dedicated to
My Late Parents
(Smt. Ramwati Devi and Devi Ram Varshney)
Teachers and Stalwarts
of Homeopathy

Central Council for Research in Homoeopathy

New Delhi, India

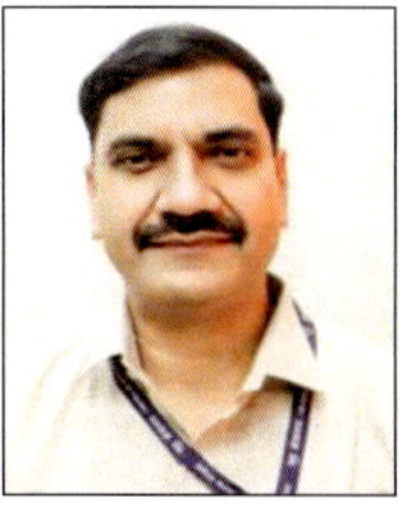

Dr. Subhash Kaushik
Director General

Foreword

In an era where veterinary medicine is advancing at an unprecedented rate, the integration of holistic approaches is becoming increasingly relevant. Homeopathy, with its rich history and unique philosophy, offers a valuable perspective in the treatment of animals. This book represents a bridge between traditional veterinary practice and alternative therapies, inviting both veterinarians and curious newcomers to explore the benefits of homeopathic medicine in this field. It provides not only a comprehensive introduction to Homeopathy but also practical guidance on its application in veterinary practice.

The author, with his extensive experience and passion for integrative medicine, offers a well-rounded view of Homeopathy's potential to enhance animal health. He has meticulously outlined the principles, remedies, and case studies that highlights the effectiveness of this approach. His insights are grounded in both scientific inquiry and clinical practice, making this book a valuable resource for those seeking to expand their understanding of veterinary homeopathy.

This book encourages veterinarians and would help researchers as a viable and compassionate option. The chapter on "Homeopathic prescribing in animals" holds immense importance for veterinarians and researchers in understanding the pet behaviour and prescribing the homeopathic similimum. Few topics like description of remedies in veterinary homeopathy book, difference between human and animal mental symptoms, prevention of diseases by homeopathic drugs other than nosodes, are noteworthy for their groundbreaking analysis, offering new perspectives that will inspire readers and motivates them to embrace a more holistic perspective that aligns with the innate healing abilities of animals.

I am assured that this book will serve as a beacon for those interested in integrating Homeopathy into their veterinary practice and validation of these clinical gems can be undertaken in research.

Dated 4th September, 24

(Subhash Kaushik)

Preface

By and large animal health care, throughout the world, is being provided by the veterinarians trained in Allopathic system of medicine as veterinary courses are available only in modern system of medicine. Philosophy of Allopathy, both in human and veterinary health care, has been widely accepted owing to discoveries of pathogen as a cause of disease; prevention of infectious diseases by antitoxins and vaccines; and antibiotics in controlling infections. Ever increasing cost of allopathic medicines has made their rational dosing in animals unaffordable to marginal farmers or landless laborers involved in unorganized animal husbandry. Injudicious, erratic and unnecessary use of antibiotics in humans and animals has given birth to the problem of microbial resistance and antimicrobial residues in animal products causing a great concern all over the world. During recent years, an interest is being invoked in seeking an alternate health care approach both in humans and animals. Homeopathy, an integral component of holistic medicine, has emerged as widely accepted complementary and alternative health care system not only in humans but also in animals because of its minimum doses, affordable cost, eco- friendliness, safety, non-toxic nature, simplicity and tailor made individualized approach. As no system of medicine is complete in itself, a holistic approach incorporating all reasonable forms of treatment appears to be more pragmatic in alleviating the sufferings of animals.

Homeopathy, conceived in 1796 by Dr. Samuel Hahnemann, originated in Germany as a unique approach to treat diseases based on the philosophy of "*Similia similibus curantur*". The founder of Homeopathy referred to the great similarity of the method as applied to animals and humans. Use of homeopathy to treat animal diseases has been a tradition almost as long as human homeopathy. Despite teething trouble such as adapting the patient questioning technique, lack of subjective symptoms and expression of emotions in animals, homeopathy has continued its place as an alternative treatment approach in the disease management of the animals.

Presently homeopathic treatment of animals is being practiced by unqualified homeopaths (farmers themselves or veterinarians trained in modern medicine) in different parts of the world extrapolating the information available in human homeopathy. Their results are highly variable and not flawless owing to casual and erratic practice based on inadequate and unqualified knowledge of homeopathy. No doubt, not much proving has been done on animals and qualified information on the use of homeopathic drugs in particular animal disease (with its detailed symptomology) is also very much restricted.

To adopt homeopathy in animal prescribing, there is a genuine need to equip veterinarians with fundamental knowledge of homeopathy; its philosophy; posology; Materia Medica; case taking; analysis and evaluation of symptoms; understanding animal constitution, psychology and behavior; homeopathic prescribing and case management. Whatever information on the use of homeopathy in animals is available is based mostly on human homeopathic Materia Medica. Recognizing the need of veterinarians for qualified homeopathic information, Veterinary Council of India has included the homeopathy in the syllabus of B.V.Sc. and A.H.course It is heartening that post graduate certificate course in Veterinary Homeopathy has also been started to make veterinarians familiar with veterinary homeopathy at Kerala Veterinary and Animal Science University and at Guru Angad Dev Veterinary and Animal Science University, Ludhiana.

At present veterinary students and veterinarians in India are not well versed with the basics and intricacies of Homeopathy to undertake the practice of homeopathy in animals on sound footing because of their no homeopathic back ground and dearth of a simplified illustrative information.

The book "**Homeopathy in Veterinary Medicine**" is an attempt to bridge the gap and has been designed as per syllabus of Veterinary Council of India. It is anticipated that the book will be helpful to veterinary students as well as practicing veterinarians who are inclined to opt for inclusion of homeopathy as an alternative, add on or exclusive therapy in their clinical practice.

J.P. Varshney

Acknowledgements

The challenge of writing a book on Homeopathy in Veterinary Medicine would not have been possible without the patience, encouragement, moral and emotional support and unbounded love of my family. Thank you very much to my better half Jai Prabha Varshney; daughters Pratibha, Ritu and Prabhanshi; sons Atul, Prabhat and Ajit; and grandchildren Agrima, Vedaant, Devansh and Anvi.

Thank you Dr. Shivang Swaminarayan for introducing me to Homeopathy. Help rendered by Dr. Hardik Monapara and Dr. Deep Bhanderi during critical times is duly acknowledged. I am grateful for the all-time support of Shri Nayan N. Bharatia, Managing trustee and Board of Trustees, Nandini Veterinary Hospital, Surat.

Thanks are also due to Dr. Ritika Hassija Narula, Research Officer, CCRH, New Delhi for her keen interest in veterinary homeopathy.

J.P. Varshney

Contents

List of Abbreviations

@	At the rate of
AAHP	American Association of Homeopathic Pharmacists
AHVMA	American Holistic Veterinary Medical Association
AI	Artificial Insemination
ALT	Alanine aminotransferase or Alanine transaminase
AST	Aspartate aminotransferase or Aspartate transaminase
BAHVS	British Association of Homeopathic Veterinary Surgeons
BID	" bis in die"(Latin) means twice daily
Bpm	Beats per minute
BUN	Blood urea nitrogen
B.V.Sc. & A.H.	Bachelor of Veterinary Science and Animal Husbandry
°C	Degree centigrade
C	Centesimal scale
CH	Centesimal dilution using Hahnemann (H) dilution method
CMT	California Mastitis Test
CNS	Central Nervous System
dl	Deciliter
DNS	Dextrose Normal Saline
E.coli	Escherichia coli
°F	Fahrenheit
FDA	Food and Drug Administration
Fig.	Figure
fT3	free- Triiodothyronine
fT4	free- thyroxine
g	gram
g-GT	gamma-glutamyl transferase
Hb	Hemoglobin
HPCUS	Homeopathic Pharmacopeia Convention of the United States
HPF	High Power Field
IAVH	International Association for Veterinary Homeopathy
i.e.	id est (that is)
IV	Intravenous
Kg	Kilogram
L	Liter
M	Roman numerical used to denote 1000 c (centesimal potency)
Mg	Milligram
µl	Micro-liter
pH	Potential of Hydrogen
%	Percent
PO	Per Os (orally)
RBC	Red blood cells (Erythrocytes)
Rs	Rupees (Indian)
SAP	Serum Alkaline Phosphatase
STT	Schirmer Tear Test

TID	"ter in die"(Latin) means three times daily
TLC	Total Leucocyte Count
U	Unit
UK	United kingdom
USA	United States of America
V/V	Volume/volume
V/W	Volume/weight
Viz.	Videre licet (Latin phrase) meaning that is to say
WBC	White Blood cells
WHO	World Health Organization

List of Figures

1

Homeopathy and Developments

Homeopathy

The word 'Homeopathy' is derived from two Greek words "Homeos" and "Pathos" meaning "similar" and "suffering" respectively (Mukherjee and Wahile,2006). This system of medicine is based on the principle of 'Similars' propounded by Dr. Samuel Hahnemann in late 17th century. The practice of Homeopathy came into being and gained wide spread popularity too early in the history of medicine at a time when it was impossible to provide any kind of explanation for its clinical efficacy. It is a complete and separate approach to health care using dynamized micro doses of herbs, minerals or animal products to stimulate the body's innate healing mechanism. Homeopathy is claimed to be more ecological, compassionate and comprehensive owing to use of micro doses. Clinical anecdotal evidence exists to indicate that homeopathy is beneficial in veterinary practice also. The homeopathic remedies stimulate the body defense to heal itself. The practice of homeopathy began first and science in its efficacy is being discovered later as was in case of immunology. An increasing interest is being shown in Homeopathy as a complementary and alternative treatment for both human and animal diseases owing to ever increasing problem of emergence of resistance in micro-organisms to antibiotics, their residues in animal products, and side effects of modern drugs. But critics of homeopathy are not reconciling with the use of highly diluted homeopathic remedies and considering it as a controversial therapy. Researches with the help of modern technology are now illustrating science in homeopathy.

Uniqueness of Homeopathy

Homeopathic drugs are considered unique owing to very minute doses of the drugs because of potentization and succussion. Decimal and Centesimal scales of potency are used. The drugs are considered non-toxic. The homeopathic therapy is tailor made individualized therapy.

Inclination towards Homeopathy

Veterinary medicine has followed in the footsteps of Human medicine. High cost of the allopathic medicines, their inherited side effects and problem of antimicrobial residues in animal products have caused an apparent discomfort to animal owners invoking their interest in alternative approaches of animal health care. Further unorganized animal sector, particularly in the hands of poor marginal farmers or landless laborers below poverty line, urges for cheaper, ecofriendly, safe and effective alternative animal health care approach as a first line therapy. Amongst alternative approaches, Homeopathy is widely accepted as a complementary and alternative approach and is probably in vogue for around 200 years. It is being practiced in the countries of the European Union and in USA also. European Union committee has also urged recently to cut the use of antimicrobials in human as well as veterinary practice to an essential level for maintaining the effectiveness of antimicrobials and to deal with the problems of emergence of resistance among microbes. Recently Americans are also inclined to encourage the use of homeopathic drugs in the management of animal diseases. The Indian scenario is also no way different. In this country many veterinarians are using homeopathic drugs in the management of animal diseases, though lacking in proper planning and execution that makes the claim of miracle cure unacceptable.

Homeopathy a Placebo or Science

Because of high dilutions exceeding Avogadro's number (6.023×10^{-23}) i.e. $\geq$12 C ,wherein there is remote chances of containing a molecule or atom of the original compound, opponents of homeopathy had been equivocal in saying that homeopathic drugs do not have more than a placebo effect. With any medical therapy there is likely to be some degree of placebo effect whether it is allopathy, homeopathy or any other kind of therapy. But arguments that the effects of Homeopathy are only a placebo response are not supported by scientific evidence. If it is just a placebo effect how does one explain the results of positive high quality placebo controlled trials, results of laboratory experiment (frog, wheat plant , leucocytes) and rigorous research studies on the effect of homeo drugs in the prevention of *E.coli* diarrhea in piglets. The basis of the placebo effect in people is experiencing a beneficial effect, arising from belief in the treatment, and based partly on confidence derived from consultations, leading to expectations on the part of the patient.

Analogy between Homeopathy and Immunology

The birth of Immunology and Homeopathy took place at the end of the eighteenth century at the same time when Jenner gave first smallpox vaccination and German physician Samuel Hahnemann was conducting his first homeopathic 'proving'. The profound analogies between homeopathic principles and immunology are due to the fact that the both are based on the principle of regulating endogenous systems of healing and its neuroendocrine integrations. Jenner's discovery of anti-small pox vaccination remained isolated episode in medicine until Pasteur connected its origin with a principle that cannot be better characterized than by Hahnemann's word: Homeopathic (Behring,1915).Around the end of 19th century Schulz and Arndt developed a principle that described that weak stimuli slightly increase biological responses, medium stimuli markedly raise them, strong ones suppress them and very strong ones arrest them. Similar observations are also seen in modern medicine. It is apparent that immunology and modern biology can offer a considerable contribution to the understanding of Homeopathy in a frame work that is not very different from the conventional one.

How homeopathic drugs act?

For long, the mechanism of action of homeopathic drugs remained obscure and it was postulated that these medicines are energy medicine and Chaos theory (Gleck, 1987) where it was assumed that minute changes can lead to huge difference; and Resonance theory where it was considered that the water, in which most of the homeopathic medicines are made, not only store frequencies (Endler, 1994) but also some form of memory, were suggested. These theories have not been substantiated experimentally. However, with advancement in molecular technology, many explanations are being postulated and it has been convincingly proved that homeopathic medicines are nano medicines and work by identification of work targets, the means of drug-receptor interactions, the mechanism of signal transmission and amplification, and the models of inversion of effects according to the traditional "smile" rule (Bellavite, 2015). Another team of scientist led by Dr. A.R. Khuda Bukhsh has provided convincing evidence of potentized homeopathic drugs' ability to trigger favourable regulatory changes in gene expression, possibly through epigenetic modifications (Khuda Bukhsh ,2015).

Benefits of integrating Homeopathy in Animal Health care

1. To some extent use of antibiotics can be reduced
2. Cost of treatment can be reduced
3. Can be used as 1st aid treatment in remote places
4. Can be used as low cost supportive therapy in some diseases.

History and Developments of Homeopathy

- Homeopathy is a system of medical practice that originated with the pioneering work of the great German physician Dr. Samuel Hahnemann (1755-1843). He discovered that patients with certain diseases could be cured with substances that produce similar toxic effects, e.g. cholera could be cured with a dose of arsenic, scarlet fever with a dose of belladonna etc. He termed this principle 'similia similibus curentur' – 'let likes be cured by likes', also known as 'similia principle' or 'law of similars'.

- Although the ancient Greek physician Hippocrates – the founder of western medicine – was the first one to moot the idea of curing 'like with like' more than 2,000 years ago, it was Hahnemann who made this principle into a system of treatment.
- Hahnemann continued to experiment with various substances, first on himself, then on other people. He soon realized that substances he gave to his patients were often toxic. He then started experimenting with diluting his formulas and discovered that the substances with more dilutions were more effective. This was his 2nd fundamental law known as the "law of infinitesimals". He diluted the preparations to an astonishing extent (1: 100000000) and insisted that homeopathic medicines retained their power provided you shook the preparation violently during the process of dilution. This process he termed as "Potentization". In 1828 he announced that all or nearly all chronic diseases were caused by the "itch" (scabies).
- In 19th century in America ,"regular" medicine was *terrible* as germ theory was still in its infancy (no vaccinations, no antibiotics, etc.). Many physicians adhered to medical theories that dated back to antiquity and employed "heroic" medical treatments (heavy bloodletting, purges, and large doses of poisonous concoctions of mercury or arsenic). Homeopathy, on the other hand, was a promising new development because of its use in small doses, its emphasis on the curative power of nature, and its holistic treatment of the body. Homeopathy started developing into a practice.
- While homeopathic medicine originated in Germany, by the 1840s the practice was flourishing in the United States. Homeopathy was just one of several sects of alternative medicine (hydropathy, osteopathy, eclectic medicine, Thomsonain medicine, and Christian Science) that emerged during this period. It was homeopathy that became biggest rival of the regular medicine. Hans Gram, a Dutch homeopath, immigrated to the USA in 1825. With his settling in America, Homeopathy took rapid strides there. Homeopathy had a large impact on the practice of medicine. The first homeopathic hospital opened in 1832 and homeopathic medical schools opened all over Europe.
- In 1844 first American Institute of Homeopathy was established. Homeopathy had a large impact on the practice of medicine.

- Throughout the 19th century, dozens of homeopathic institutions appeared in Europe and the United States.
- In 1846-1847, the American Medical Association was founded, largely as an effort to expel homeopaths from the profession and the last traditional homeopathic college closed its doors in the 1920s. Revival of homeopathy took place in America in 1960s and 1970s.
- While traditional homeopathic practice largely faded away by mid-century, the sketchiest part of homeopathy — those vials of diluted nothingness — survived. In 1938 the FDA passed the Federal Food, Drug, and Cosmetic Act (FD&C Act), which included a section that recognized homeopathic medicines and appointed a non-governmental body, the Homeopathic Pharmacopeia Convention of the United States (HPCUS), responsible for establishing safety and manufacturing guidelines.
- Homeopathy was revived in 20th century.
- In the 21st century, criticism for homeopathy was renewed as a series of meta-analyses have shown that the treatment results claimed with homeopathy lack scientific justification. As a result, national and international bodies have recommended the withdrawal of government funding for homeopathy in healthcare. National bodies from Australia, United Kingdom, Switzerland and France, as well as the European Academies' Science Advisory Council and the Russian Academy of Sciences have all concluded that homeopathy is ineffective, and recommended against the practice receiving any further funding. The National Health Service in England stopped funding for homeopathic remedies. France also stopped funding in 2021. Spain also announced to ban homeopathy from health centers.

Homeopathy around the World Today

- Despite countless barriers, popularity of homeopathy is growing today throughout the world.
- It is much popular in Asia, from Pakistan, Bangladesh, Nepal , Sri Lanka to India
- In India, homeopathy is officially recognized as a separate branch of the medicine and is flourishing with full support of the government.
- India has the largest number of homeopathic hospitals in the world, over 100,000 homeopathic doctors, and over 120 homeopathic colleges.

- Homeopathy is also becoming popular throughout Europe. In England, France, and Germany, with the availability of homeopathic medicines in most pharmacies.
- In England, homeopathic hospitals were opened in Bristol, Liverpool, Glasgow, Tunbridge Wells, and London throughout the late nineteenth and early twentieth century. In 1948, homeopathy was incorporated into the National Health Service as an officially approved method of treatment.
- Homeopathy has become more wide spread over the past decade in many other nations, including Australia, New Zealand, South Africa, Israel, and Greece. In addition, homeopathy is highly respected in many South American countries, especially Mexico, Argentina, and Brazil.
- Presently many courses are offered in veterinary homeopathy in Great Britain, Holland and Germany. In USA, the Academy Of Veterinary Homeopathy offers courses in veterinary classical homeopathy. In 1986 veterinarians from Belgium, Germany, Great Britain, Italy, France, Luxembourg and the Netherlands founded the International association for veterinary homeopathy (IAVH) in Luxembourg

History of Homeopathy in India

- History of homeopathy in India dates back to as early as 1810 when, Dr. John Martin Honigberger, a disciple of Dr. Samuel Hahnemann , visited India and treated patients.
- In 1839, Dr. John Martin Honigberger treated Maharaja Ranjit Singh, the then ruler of Punjab, with homeopathic *Dulcamara* for paralysis of vocal cord and edema. Later he continued his homeopathic practice in Calcutta for some times.
- Homeopathy flourished in Bengal at first, then spread to other parts of India.
- In the beginning homeopathy was practiced by amateurs in civil and military services.
- Dr. Mahendra Lal Sircar was the first Indian who became homeopathic physician. Many other allopathic doctors started homeopathic practice.
- The ancient Hindu physicians had, in fact recognized the “Law of Similars” as one of the principles of treatment. Surgeon Samuel Brooking, a retired Medical Officer had the courage and conviction to establish a Homoeoapthic Hospital at Tanjore, in South India, in 1847.
- In 1881 first homeopathic college was established in Calcutta.

- Official recognition began with the passing of the first resolution by the government in 1937, followed by another in 1948. But it was only in 1952 that homeopathy began gaining recognition in the states.
- In 1973, a Central Act was passed, recognizing this system of medicine. Since its constitution in 1973, the Central Council of Homoeopathy has set minimum standards of education related to graduate and postgraduate courses and only approved colleges can provide education in homeopathy
- Today, homeopathy is a part of the national network of health services, through hospitals, dispensaries and private practitioners. "Today there are 186 degree colleges. India has the largest pool of homeopaths (2,40,000) in the world.

History and Development of Veterinary Homeopathy

- A German physician Dr Samuel Hahnemann, who first experimented on himself to test the drug- China discovered homeopathy in Germany. He then propounded the law of "Similia Similibus Curentus". He noticed that the drugs in pure form in healthy persons produce an adverse reaction resulting in symptoms of illness but the same drug in potentized form had a tremendous ability to cure the symptoms caused by the drug in pure form.
- History of veterinary homeopathy also dates back to the inception of homeopathy.
- Hahnemann himself wrote and spoke of the use of homeopathy in animals other than humans.
- In 1813 in Leipzig, Hahnemann lectured on the use of homeopathy in animals and stated that the principles and application in animals were broadly similar to those in humans.
- Boenninghausen and Lux were early proponents of homeopathy in animals. Boenninghausen, the German baron, lawyer and agriculturalist, used homoeopathy on animals and established the principles of Veterinary Homeopathy. An early advocate of high potencies, he conducted a successful prospective trial of 200C potency in domestic animals, reasoning that veterinary homeopathy was a good way to demonstrate that it was not a placebo.
- Veterinary homeopathy has a tradition almost as long as Human Homeopathy. It is evident from the literature that a German practitioner Guillaume Lux was using homeopathic drugs (*Aconitum napellus,*

Camphora, Nux vomica and *opium*) for the treatment of certain diseases of horses and cattle as early as 1833.

- Homeopathic treatment of animals was introduced by Baron Von Boenninghausen (Boger, 1938) who treated various species of animals using homeopathic drugs and established the principles of veterinary homeopathy. Since then veterinary homeopathy has continued to develop despite the apparent difficulty of lack of expression of subjective feeling in animals .It has its strongest modern tradition in Europe particularly in Germany, France and Great Britain. Macleod practiced veterinary homeopathy from World War II until his death in 1995. In the UK there are many vets practicing homoeopathy and over one third of these have qualified to the Faculty Homeopathy's MF Hom Vet level. Their interest is maintained by the British Association of Homoeopathic Veterinary Surgeons (BAHVS). By 1906, Humphrey's company was producing a range of homeopathic remedies for veterinary use.
- Presently many courses are offered in veterinary homeopathy in Great Britain, Holland and Germany. In USA, the Academy Of Veterinary Homeopathy offers courses in veterinary classical homeopathy. In 1986 veterinarians from Belgium, Germany, Great Britain, Italy, France, Luxembourg and the Netherlands founded the International Association for Veterinary Homeopathy (IAVH) in Luxembourg.
- Tradition of veterinary homeopathy is as old as humans. Initially homeopathic drugs viz. Aconitum napellus, Camphora, Nux vomica and Opium were being used for the treatment of certain diseases of horses and cattle as early as 1833 by German Practitioner – Guillaume Lux. Since then veterinary homeopathy has progressed considerably despite the apparent difficulty in adopting the patient questioning technique, lack of expression of subjective feelings and lack of experimental data. Published reports on the use of homeopathic drugs in animal health care has done little to convince veterinarians trained in modern medicine possibly due to inappropriate research procedures to satisfy a modern veterinarian. This necessitates further research satisfying both the basic tenets of homeopathy as well as allopathy. Animal experimentation is a well accepted research tool in modern medicine. Double blind, cross-over trials are also bastion of modern scientific clinical trial. Unfortunately neither of these methodologies is appropriate to homeopathy. What is needed is a large scale clinical trial under field conditions. Wherein at least disease diagnosis is based on sound scientific footings including history, clinical manifestations, laboratory investigations, electrocardiography, ultrasonography, radiography and / or endoscopy as the case may be.

- In 2016, a review of peer-reviewed articles (from 1981 to 2014) by scientists from the University of Kassel, Germany, concluded that there is lack of scientific evidence to support homeopathy as an effective treatment of infectious diseases in livestock. The UK's Department for Environment, Food and Rural Affairs also showed disapproval for the use of homeopathy. The British Veterinary Association has also taken a stand not to endorse homeopathy. The Australian Veterinary Association has included homeopathy on its list of "ineffective therapies.
- Despite lack of ideal research programs , clients as well as veterinarians in many countries including India are convinced of the value of homeopathy. Nevertheless, proper scientific proving will be the only route to consistent success and ethical practice of homeopathy in veterinary medicine. It is hoped that more and more scientific approach will help to optimize the use homeo drugs in veterinary practice.

History of Veterinary homeopathy in India

- In India veterinary homeopathy is being practiced by amateurs, farmers and veterinarians having no authenticated basic scientific knowledge of homeopathy.
- There are many scattered case reports on the use of homeo drugs in the treatment of animal ailments with variable protocol and results lacking uniformity.
- There is no doubt on professional acumen; nevertheless, their practice of homeopathy is not flawless owing to lack of planning and proper execution. The practices seem casual and erratic lacking scientific fervor owing to unconfirmed diagnoses, no laboratory substantiation, improper follow up observations and lack of documentary evidences.
- Large scale clinical trials based on scientific lines are entirely lacking.
- Scientific validation of homeopathic drugs in the treatment of animal diseases in modern perspective will not only make veterinarians far more confident in adopting homeopathy as an efficacious cost effective therapeutic and/ or preventive modality of animal health care but also diffuse the apprehension of its folksy and wired system of esoteric medicine. Before 2001 no planned research project was undertaken to evaluate homeopathic drugs in the treatment of animal diseases anywhere in the country because of lack of confidence of veterinarians, trained in modern medicine, on the efficacy of homeopathic drugs. Recognizing the need of reducing the use of antibiotics in animal treatment and having a cheap and effective alternative medicine

(as a first line therapy that may be used by farmers in remote places) a project entitled "Evaluation of Homeopathic Drugs in the Management of Animal Diseases" was conceived and initiated in December. 2001 in the Division of Medicine with collaboration of Division of Surgery and Division of Animal Reproduction, Indian Veterinary Research Institute, Izatnagar, Bareilly. Both concepts of individual drug and homeopathic combination remedy were put to trial in diseases of large animals and companion animals with confirmed diagnoses based on modern diagnostic techniques. The encouraging results of the validation studies led to the publication of a book entitled" Research Findings: Homeopathic Bioefficacy and Management of Animal Health " edited by Dr.J.P.Varshney (then Principal Scientist, Division Of Veterinary Medicine, Indian Veterinary Research Institute, Izatnagar, Bareilly, U.P) and Dr. Shivang Swaminarayan (then Head of Health Care Division, Sintex International Limited, Kalol, Ahmedabad) in year 2007.

- Later Central Council for research in Homeopathy (CCRH, New delhi), Govt.of India started encouraging research in veterinary homeopathy by funding research projects in veterinary institutes/ universities.
- At present there is no association of veterinarians practicing homeopathy in India. Whatever is being practiced in veterinary homeopathy has been borrowed from human homeopathy. Specialized courses to train veterinarians in homeopathy in India had remained non- existent till 2015.
- Despite absence of veterinary homeopathy forum in India , reluctance of veterinarians trained in modern system of medicine to accept findings of homeopathic trials in animals and general apathy, clinical research findings of homeopathic remedies in animals have been disseminated to sensitize practicing veterinarians through National and International forums of Human Homeopathy and Veterinary (Varshney and Kumar, 2003, Banyopadhyay and Varshney, 2004, Bandyopadhyay and Varshney, 2005, Varshney and Saghar, 2005, Varshney, 2005 a, Chinkija and Varshney, 2005 b, Swaminarayan and Varshney, 2010, Varshney and Swaminarayan 2010 a and b, Varshney and Swaminarayan 2011 a and b, Varshney, 2011 a and b, Varshney and Swaminarayan, 2014, Varshney, 2015, Varshney, 2016 a, Varshnety and Swaminarayan, 2018) and other national and international scientific forums (Ram Naresh *et al.*, 2002, Varshney, 2003, Kumar *et al.*, 2003, Varshney and Ram Naresh, 2003, Kumar *et al.*, 2004, Varshney and Kumar, 2004, Swaminarayan and Varshney, 2005, Kumar and Varshney 2005, Varshney, 2005 b,

Varshney, 2005 c, Chinkija and Varshney, 2005 a, Varshney *et al.*, 2007, Varshney, 2013 a).

- In academic year 2015-16, Kerala Veterinary and Animal Science University took the lead to start a Post graduate certificate course in Veterinary Homeopathy (Directorate of Academics and Research No. KVASU/DAR/Acad (B 1)/ 1 397 7 12014 (15.4's) Dated, Pookode, 05/03/201 5).
- Very recently in 2024 Guru Angad Dev Veterinary and Animal Science University, Ludhiana has also initiated an Online Post graduate certificate course in Veterinary Homeopathy.

References and Literature Reviewed

Ajay Kumar and Varshney, J.P. (2005). A preliminary study on antihaemorrhagic efficacy of a homeo-complex in the management of hemorrhagic crisis in dogs. Natn. Seminar Homeopathic medicine Plant Animals and Fishes, Thrissur, 5-6th February, 05, p.79.

Behring, E.(1915). Gesammelte Abhandlungen. Neue Folge. Bonn: Marcus and Weber, 1915.

Bellavite, P.(2015). Hypothesis and findings on the action mechanism(s) of homeopathic drugs. GHF's World Homeopathy Summit on Recent Advances in Scientific Research. Birla Matushree Sabhaghar, Mumbai, 11-12th Aprol, 2015.

Changkija, B. and Varshney, J.P. (2005). Effect of Abies nigra on heart rate and rhythm in tachycardimic dogs- A case study. International Homeopathic Conference, Toronto, Canada, October 22-23, 05.

Endler, P.C.(1994).The effect of highly diluted agitated thyroxine on the climbing activity of frogs. Vet.Hum. Toxicol 36:56.

Gleck, J.(1987). Chaos, Newyork, Penguin.

Harendra Kumar,Srivastava,S.K.,Yadav, M.C. and Varshney, J.P (2003). Management of post-partum anestrus in dairy animals with a homeopathic combination remedy.Nat.Symp. Challenges Strategies Sust. Anim.Prod. in Mountains, Palampur, 14th-15th April,2003.

Khuda Bukhsh, A.R. (2015). An evidence-based gene regulatory hypothesis to explain molecular mechanism of action of potentized homeopathic drugs in all living organisms. GHF's World Homeopathy Summit on Recent Advances in Scientific research. Birla Matushree Sabhaghar, Mumbai, 11-12th April, 2015.

Mukherjee, P.K.and Wahile, A.(2006). Integrated approaches towards drug development from Ayurveda and other Indian system of medicines. J. Ethnopharmacol. 103:25-35.

Raj Kumar, R., Srivastava, S.K., Yadav, M.C., Harendra Kumar, Varshney, V.P. and Varshney, J.P. (2004).Effect of homeopathic combination remedy on estrus induction and hormonal profile in anestrus cows. XX Annual Convention of ISSAR and National Symposium, Durg, 14th –16th Dec.,2004, pp 39-40.

Ram Naresh, Varshney, J.P. and Mukherjee, Reena (2002). Management of udder affections with homeopathic formulation – a preliminary trial. 10th International Congress AAAP, NewDelhi, 23rd-27th \ September,2002.

Varshney, J.P., Deshmukh,V.V.and Chaudhary, P.S. (2007). Clinical Management of common cold in a Labrador pup with Allium cepa 30C.. 15th All India Homeopathic Scientific Seminar, Rajkot, 21-23rd Dec., 2007.

Varshney, J.P. (2003). Evaluation of a homeopathic combination remedy in the Management of canine viral gastroenteritis simulating to parvo. Natn. Symp. Focussing Need Develop

New Diag.Therap. Prev. Approaches Deal Disorders farm Comp.Anims. Anand, 7th-9th February, 2003.

Varshney, J.P. (2004). Management of pyrexia in animals with homeopathic drug. World Herbo Expo-2004, Bhopal, 12th-14th January, 2004.

Varshney, J.P. (2005 a). Hepatoprotective efficacy of a homeopathic combination remedy in phenobarbital induced hepatopathy in epileptic dogs. Natn.Seminar Homeopathic Medicine Plant, Animals and Fishes, Thrissur,5-6th February, 05,pp1-5.

Varshney, J.P. (2005b). Prospects of Homeopathy in Veterinary Medicine in India. National Workshop under ASCAD on use of Alternative Systems of Medicine (Ayurvedic and Homeopathic) in Veterinary Practice, Nagpur, May 5-6, 05, pp 14-19.

Varshney, J.P. (2005c). Reversal of paroxysmal atrial tachycardia with oral administration of Digitalis 6C in dogs. International conference on "Actual points for Veterinary Homeopathy", St.Petersburg, Russia, December 20-24, 2005.

Varshney, J.P. (2011).An overview of Research in Homeopathic Veterinary Medicine in India. Liga 2011 Varshney, J.P.(2011). Diagnosis and Management of Atrial Paroxysmal Tachycardia in Dogs with Homeopathic Digitalis. Liga 2011

Varshney, J.P. and Ajay Kumar (2003). Management of pyrexia syndrome with a homeopathic combination remedy. 14th International Homeopathic Congress. 17th -19th October,2003, New Delhi, India.

Varshney, J.P. and Ajay Kumar (2004). Clnical management of epilepsy in dogs with homeopathic drugs. Natn.Symp. Latest Approaches Biotech.Tools Hlth.Manage.Farm Comp.Anims., Izatnagar, 11th-13th February, 2004.

Varshney, J.P. and Ram Naresh (2003). Management of udder affections of Indian buffaloes with a homeopathic combination remedy. 4th Asian Buffalo Congress, NewDelhi, 25th-28th February, 2003.

Varshney, J.P. and Saghar, S.Soja (2005). Evaluation of hepatoprotective efficacy of a homeo-complex in dogs with hepatopathy. International Conference on "Actual points for Veterinary Homeopathy", St. Petersburg, Russia, December 20-24, 2005.

Varshney, J.P.and Swaminarayan, S.(2010). Homeopathic drugs in the management of anaemia in animals. Brain Storming Session at CFTRI, MysoreVarshney, J.P. and Swaminarayan, S, (2010). Clinical management of gastroenteritis with Arsenic album 30C in animals. XXII National Congress of Indian Institute of Homeopathic Physicians, Delhi State Branch, Delhi.

Varshney, J.P. and Swaminarayan, S. (2011) Clinical Management of Thelitis with homeopathic drugs in cows and buffaloes. Liga 2011.

Varshney, J.P. and Swaminarayan, S. (2018). Case Study: Canine Bladder Tumour (Transitional Cell Carcinoma). 3rd International Conference on Integrative Oncology. Nashik (19-21 Jan, 2018).

Varshney, J.P. nd Swaminarayan, S.(2011). Clinical Management of Gastroenteritis with Arsenic album 30C in animals Asian Conference held at Ceylon.

2

Basic Principles and Philosophy of Homeopathy

Homeopathy

Homeopathy is a different system of health care being practiced across the world. It is not only an alternate health approach but a distinct full-fledged complete rational system of medicine having holistic, individualistic, and dynamistic approach to life, health, disease, remedy and cure. This system of health care science is offering treatment option for acute and chronic ailments of humans and animals. Homoeopathy takes a holistic approach towards the sick individual through promotion of inner balance at mental, emotional, spiritual and physical levels.

Birth of Homeopathy

Homeopathy was founded by Dr Hahnemann who was more concerned to evolve a safe and effective therapeutic paradigm around the key concept of similia. Dr. Hahnemann codified a new medical system with seven principles/ concepts when vital force theory , miasmatic theory of causation of diseases (Bhalwar, 2009) were prevalent and the concept of drug proving on healthy human being was proposed by Albrecht von Haller (Hahnemann,1922) .He fortified his key concept of "similia" with drug proving, drug dynamisation and individualization, and four ancillary theories viz. chronic diseases (Miasm), vital force (vital principle), single medicine and minimum dose. He named his new system of therapy as "Homeopathy" and published the first edition of Organon of Medicine in 1810.

Basic Principles of Homeopathy

Dr. Hahnemann, the Father of Homeopathy, propounded the new system of health care, named as the Homeopathy, with seven basic concepts.

- Law of Similia
- Law of Simplex
- Law of Minimum

- Doctrine of Drug Proving
- Theory of chronic Diseases
- Theory of Vital Force
- Doctrine of Drug Dynamization

Law of Similia

Key concept of homeopathy is "similia similibus curantur" or "Like cures like" that was known in medicine from the time of Hippocrates or even in the ancient Indian system of Ayurveda. This first concept was proposed for Homeopathy by Hahnemann in 1796. The principle of similia similibus curantur (Latin phrase) is one of the pillars of the homeopathic doctrine established by Samuel Hahnemann. The meaning of the Latin phrase is that " like is cured by like":i.e. the disease may be cured by something that can cause similar symptoms. This law states that a drug, capable of producing a diseased-state in a healthy person or individual exactly similar to that observed in a diseased person, acts as a therapeutic agent if the disease is in a curable stage. In the incurable stage of the disease, however, the same drug acts as the best palliative. Hahnemann postulated that vast set of symptoms produced by any substance on a group of healthy individuals can be cured in a sick person by application of the same substance. A simple example of this doctrine is that of onion and *Allium cepa* (homoeopathic preparation of red onion). Peeling of onion causes watering and burning sensation in eyes and nose. According to the principle of Homoeopathy, a person suffering from similar watering and burning sensation in eyes and nose (frequently seen with common cold) can be effectively treated by the homeopathic medicine *Allium cepa*, prepared from red onion.

Law of Simplex

Hahnemann stated that only one single, simple medicinal substance should be administered in a given case at a time. Remedies were proved singly. If more than one remedy is given, pure effect of the remedy cannot be observed. According to this law, use of multiple drugs is not desirable.

Law of Minimum

Law of minimum states that the given medicine should be in a very minute dose. This can be achieved by a process of drug dynamisation or process of drug potentization. By giving minimum dose of the drug, unwanted aggression is avoided and dynamic action of the given medicine is increased. The law of minimum finds support from Arndt-Schultz law. According to that law small doses stimulate, medium doses paralyze and large doses kill.

Drug Proving

Drug proving is a systematic investigation of the pathogenetic (symptom producing) powers of the medicine on the healthy humans of different ages, sexes, and constitutions. Healthy persons volunteering for drug proving are called prover. An ideal prover should be healthy, intelligent, delicate, sensitive, truthful and unprejudiced. Drug proving on humans has an advantage of expression of subjective and mental symptoms. Action of the drugs on the healthy subjects is different from that of sick subjects. Drug proving on animals are lacking. Animals cannot express subjective symptom and expression of feelings (emotions) is absent. It is only objective symptoms in animals that makes the expression of the proving difficult.

Theory of Chronic Disease

The theory of chronic disease was added by Hahnemann in the 4th edition of Organon. He observed that inspite of best homeopathic treatment there was recurrence of chronic diseases. After his long observation he concluded that chronic diseases were due to chronic miasms. The word “Miasm” has its origin from Greek word “ Miasma” meaning a polluting agent. The chronic miasms are Psora, Sychosis and Syphilis. Psora is the fundamental cause of innumerable diseases and manifested as cutaneous itching eruptions. Syphilis, another miasm, is characterized by granulation, denegeration and ulceration. Sychosis , 3rd miasm , is characterized by cauliflower like growths (wart) on genital region, induration and infiltration.

Theory of Vital Force

Vital force which is governing the material body is single and dynamic. In Organon, Hahnemann stated that ‘In the healthy condition of the man, the spiritual vital force (autocracy), the dynamis that animate the material body (organism), rules with unbounded sway and retain all the parts of the organism in admirable, harmonious, vital operation, as regards both sensations and functions, so that our indwelling, reason-gifted mind can freely employ this living, healthy instrument for the higher purposes of our existence’. He further said that the material organism, without vital force, is capable of no sensation, no function, no self-preservation; it derives all sensation and performs all the functions of life solely by means of immaterial being (vital force) which animates the material organism in health and disease.

Drug Dynamyzation or Potentization

Another concept of Hahnemann’s new medical system was Drug dynamization (dilution with succussion) i.e. diluting the original material to reduce its toxicity. He arrived on mathematically evolved sequential dilutions of decimal, centesimal and the millismal modelling with a method of succussions/ titurations to enhance the pharamaco-dynamic properties of even inert substances. In other words the process of dynamization awakens the latent medicinal properties in natural crude substances. This concept was introduced by Hahnemann in 5th edition of Organon and it became controversial because it defied the material scientific theories (Avogadro's constant). According to this concept, there won't be any matter of the original solute beyond the 23rd decimal potency or 12th centesimal potency of homeopathic medicine. In homeopathy it is claimed that the drugs of higher dynamised potency have higher curative properties. This concept seems to be in accordance with Arndt Schulz Law that says that every substance at small doses stimulate, moderate doses inhibit and in large doses kill. The process of dynamisation has a benefit of making the deadly poisons harmless, making the medicinally inert substances in crude state active, making the action of the potentized medicines deeper and longer, and avoiding unnecessary aggravation.

Dosage of Homeopathic Drugs

Dosage of homeopathic drug is not related to body size of the animal but more to observable dynamics of the body and the disease. Therefore, amount of the drug does not matter much. The number of pilules taken in a single dose is relatively less important than the potency.

Potency of Homeopathic Drugs

Potency of the homeopathic drug is an important factor in the treatment. Potencies above than 30 centesimal are characterized as higher potency and below as lower potency. Potencies are selected on the basis of susceptibility of the patient, nature of the disease and nature of the drug, and symptoms of the drug and the patient. Lower potencies are used if focus of symptoms is physical/organic, in the beginning of treatment, in acute cases, and in conjunction with patients on conventional medicines. While higher potencies are used if emphasis of symptom is psychological, repeated at less frequency and are generally considered for chronic ailments.

Frequency of Dosing

Frequency is determined according to disease dynamic and patient response. Acute conditions require more frequent dosing than chronic ailments. In general, the drug is repeated only when the effect of the first dose has worn off and symptoms persist. As long as the patients feel comfort, there is no need to repeat the drug. Single most error in prescribing homeopathic drug is over medication.

Duration of Dosing

Duration of therapy is governed by the response of the patient. Treatment should not be given longer than necessary. It should be stopped as soon as symptoms cease to exist.

References and Literature Reviewed

Bhalwar, R.V. (2009) Text Book of Public Health & Community Medicine, 1st Edition.

Hahnemann, S. (1922) Organon of Medicine, Translated with Preface by William Boericke.

3

Organon of Medicine

Organon

Organon of Medicine, a document of Homeopathic philosophy articulated by Dr. Samuel Hahnemann, is the corner stone of Homeopathic principles and practices being followed by homeopaths throughout world. Before Organon of Medicine Dr. Hahnemann published an article "Essay on a New Principle" in 1796. The article was based on his first experience of the effect of Peruvian Bark Cinchona in 1790. The Organon of Medicine developed slowly out of Hahnemann's research and experimentation over a period of time and newer experiences were added in subsequent editions. With more personal observations and experimentation, he published his new account of Homeopathy in 1810 in the form of a book entitled "*Organon of Rational Art of Healing* (*Organon der rationellen Heilkunde*). It was the 1st edition. Dr. Hahnemann laid out the doctrine of his ideas of Homeopathy in this book. The book contains the principles and philosophical back ground of the Practice of Homeopathy. The work was repeatedly revised by him and published in six editions, with the name changed from the second edition onwards to Organon of Medicine (*Organon der Heilkunst*). The book saw its five editions in the life time of Hahnemann and the 6th edition was published long after the death of Dr. Hahnemann. The 2nd edition was published in 1819, with the revised title *Organon of Healing Art*. The 3rd edition of the book came in 1824. The 4th edition was published in 1829 and introduced Hahnemann's "Theory of Chronic Diseases". The 5th edition of the book was published in 1833, that contained the doctrine of vital force and drug-dynamization. The sixth edition, written in 1842, a year before his death, was retitled *Organon of Medicine* and published in 1921 (78 years after his death in 1843).

This sixth edition incorporates his latest findings, deemed to be most perfect, during his dying years. Many newer concepts like replacement of the vital force by vital principle, the 50 millesimal scale of potency and permissibility of external applications were introduced for the first time. High on philosophy, Footnotes explaining difficult concepts, Evolution of medical science reinstated. This edition contains his revised and reinvented thoughts clarifying many counter thoughts on 291 points. In this edition there is mention of origin of disease denying a Materia peccans, as the prime etiological agent. Another significant addition in this edition was with regards to doses in the treatment of chronic diseases. He revised the concept of single dose in chronic diseases and advocated repetition of doses but in different potencies. The concept of treatment of the chronic diseases under psora, syphilis and sycosis, advocated in previous edition, has been replaced with advocacy of commencing treatment with large doses of their specific remedies early and , if necessary, several times daily and gradually changing to higher potencies. His thoughts about healing effect of massage, lukewarm water bath, mesmerism, power of magnet, dynamic force of electricity, mineral magnets and galvanism in the 6th edition reflects his broad vision and deep understanding of the nature. This 6th edition of Organon of Medicine contains his philosophic insight in to the practice of Medicine (Boericke, 1921) and is a richest treasure of new thinking and knowledge created by a flawless experimenter (Dr. Hahnemann) far ahead of time.

Literature Reviewed

Ernst, E. (December 2012). "Homeopathy: a critique of current clinical research". Skeptical Inquirer. 36 (6).

Grimes, D.R. (2012). "Proposed mechanisms for homeopathy are physically impossible". Focus on Alternative and Complementary Therapies. 17 (3): 149–55. doi:10.1111/j.2042-7166.2012.01162.x.

"Homeopathic products and practices: assessing the evidence and ensuring consistency in regulating medical claims in the EU" (PDF). European Academies' ScienceAdvisory Council. September 2017. p. 1. Retrieved 1 October 2017. We agreewith previous extensive evaluations concluding that there are no known diseases for which there is robust, reproducible evidence that homeopathy is effective beyond the placebo effect.

"Homeopathy". American Cancer Society. Retrieved October 12, 2014.

Hahnemann, Samuel (1833). The Homœopathic Medical Doctrine, or Organon of the Healing Art. Translated by Devrient, Charles H. Notes by Stratten, Samuel. Dublin: W.F. Wakeman. OCLC 32732625. OL 6983421M. – Full text in PDF and DjVu formats.

Hahnemann, Samuel (1849). Organon of Medicine. Translated by Dudgeon, R.E. (from the Fifth German ed.). London: Headland. OCLC 679303968.

Hahnemann, Samuel (1921) Organan of Medicine. 6th edn. Translated by Boericke, Willam (1921). Jain B. Puyblishers (P) Ltd. USA-Europe-India

Hahnemann, Samuel; Hering, Constantine; Matlack, Charles F.; North American Academy of the Homoeopathic Healing Art (1836). Organon of homoeopathic medicine (First American, from the British translation of the German fourth ed.). Allentown, Pennsylvania: Academical Bookstore. OCLC 173514027.

Oliver Wendell Holmes Sr. (1842). Homoeopathy and its kindred delusions: Two lecturesdelivered before the Boston Society for the Diffusion of Useful Knowledge. Boston, as reprinted in Oliver Wendell Holmes Sr. (1861). Currents and counter-currents in medical science. Ticknor and Fields. pp. 72–188. OCLC 1544161. OL 14731800M.

Organon der rationellen Heilkunde nach homöopathischen Gesetzen, 1810. OL 24352038M.

Richard Haehl, Samuel Hahnemann His Life & Work, vol 2, p.379

Shang, Aijing; Huwiler-Müntener, Karin; Nartey, Linda; Jüni, Peter; Dörig, Stephan; Sterne, Jonathan AC; Pewsner, Daniel; Egger, Matthias (2005). "Are the clinical effects of homoeopathy placebo effects? Comparative study of placebo-controlled trials of homoeopathy and allopathy". The Lancet. 366 (9487): 726–32. doi:10.1016/S0140-6736(05)67177-2. PMID 16125589. S2CID 17939264.

Trevor Cook, Samuel Hahnemann His Life and Times, India: B Jain, 2001, p.177 External links[edit]

UK Parliamentary Committee Science and Technology Committee - "Evidence Check 2: Homeopathy"

Whitney, Jerome (2010). "The Evolution of the Organon" (PDF). ARH Journal: 21. {{cite journal}}: Cite journal requires |journal= (help)

4

Concepts in Homeopathy

The concepts of health, disease, symptoms, constitution, cure, vital force, suppression of the disease, individualization, totality of symptoms, and dose etc. are unique in homeopathy differing from concepts of modern medicine.

Health

Generally, health is considered as freedom from disease. According to World Health Organization health is "a state of complete physical, mental and social well-being, not merely the absence of disease or infirmity" (WHO, 1946). In homeopathy, it is defined as mental, physical and emotional wellbeing (Mondal, 2006 a) and the healthy body has been described as one in balance and equilibrium. The equilibrium of internal parameters is maintained by "life forces" corresponding to a general interpretation of immune system . In fact 'Life force" is the actual energy behind the biochemistry of the body. It ends with death of the organism.

Disease

Departure form anatomy and normal physiological functions of the body is termed as disease in modern science. A disease is a particular abnormal condition that adversely affects the structure or function of all or part of an organism and is not immediately due to any external injury (Wikipedia). In homeopathy, the disease is the dynamic disturbance of harmonious relation between the material body and vital force that stimulates the body in health (Mondal,2006 b). In nut shell the disease is the disturbance of the equilibrium of internal parameters of the body maintained by "Life force", The disturbance or imbalance of equilibrium may be temporary (with balance restored quickly-acute disease) or permanent (leading to chronic disease).

Symptoms

The symptoms are the result of body's fight to restore equilibrium. It means symptoms are generated by the body in its fight (defense) to regain equilibrium of internal parameters.

Constitution

Constitution is the underlying concept in homeopathy. It is the necessary perspective of the individual. In fact, Constitution is the genetic quality shown as biochemistry, physiology, and psychology, as adjusted by the present and past environmental conditions. Chronic disease affects nutritional factors, learned behavior and thought patterns, etc. These all factors become contributors in the disparities and flaws in one's constitution (Mondal,2006 c).

Cure

Cure is defined in Homeopathy as complete elimination of symptoms and even effects of other treatments. Feeling of wellbeing requiring continuous treatment is not cure but is palliation (Mondal,2006 d).

Vital Force

The vital force stimulates the material organism in health and disease. In homeopathy, the person/ animal is taken as a whole. It is assumed that entire life processes on physical, mental or psychological levels depend on the strength of the vital force (Mondal,2006 e).

Suppression of Disease

It is another concept in homeopathy that stresses on the assessment of the whole individual rather taking local complaints in a disease process. When only symptoms are treated without treating an individual as a whole, suppression of the disease takes place and its reappearance is in a more worsen form. Atopic dermatitis in dogs and cats, asthma in cats is suppressed with corticosteroid therapy.

Concept of Individualization

Homeopathy is a system that individualizes medicines as per totality of unique and idiosyncratic symptoms experienced by a patient (man or animal) and therefore can aptly be called as "Designer Medicine" or 'Tailor Made Medicine". From homeopathic point of view, disease does not exist. It is the diseased animal or diseased man that exists. The sick animals do not have a disease but have a syndrome of body-mind constellation of symptoms. The concept of individualization is an attempt to understand the patient in totality. It is crucial to diagnose the disease of the patient with a deeper understanding on his/her constitution, temperament, presenting complaints, genetic makeup, personal, past and present histories etc. This is a unique process of profiling the patient. This approach is getting more validity from the science of medicine and now a totally new field of personal medicine is emerging. With more understanding on genetics and gene expressions, the individualization is likely to get more rational position in the science of Homeopathy. It is the process of differentiating one from other. Hahnemann thought that no two individuals are same. Each individual manifest symptoms differently for a similar problem. Symptoms are divided as common and uncommon. Symptoms manifested by everyone suffering from same ailment are common symptoms. While uncommon symptoms are peculiar characteristic of an individual. The uncommon symptoms help to individualize the patient. The uncommon symptoms play vital role in homeopathic prescribing. Animals experience disease manifestations in subtly and sometimes overtly different way. Manifestations of a disease may be different in different animals. For example one animal with liver disease may show jaundice, other may show ascites, another may show anemia, or someone may show coagulopathy or hypoalbuminemia. Temperamentally one may be aggressive, other may be lethargic or another may be inattentive. One is comfortable in warm place while other is comfortable in cool place. Their thirst level may vary. Not only physical symptoms but also behavioral expression of the animals in the same disease differs making them unique individual. Homeopathy believes that sick animals have a syndrome (body mind cluster of symptoms) rather than having simply a disease. Therefore, selection of a drug in homeopathy stresses on taking an account of all these body mind cluster of symptoms.

Concept of Totality of Symptoms

Health is a condition of life where there is a harmonious play of vital force. Whereas disease is a condition of discomfort where harmony of vital force is disturbed and reflected through the symptoms. It is outwardly reflection of internal essence of the disease. The totality of individual symptoms includes location, sensation, modalities and concomitant. The totality of symptoms constitutes subjective symptoms, objective symptoms, those enquired from bystanders. To ensure cure totality of symptoms must be removed. Dr. Hahnemann observed that the best results of the treatment were obtained when the symptoms obtained from the proving of a medicine matched completely with the symptoms of the patient, not just the presenting signs. So it is important to take into account other symptoms also besides the prominent presenting signs. In homeopathy such other additional symptoms are known as 'concomitants. Symptoms pertaining to physical condition are termed as 'local or particular' symptom. Symptoms such as appetite, craving for particular food, effect of heat and cold or related to weather change are also required to be taken into cognizance for a successful homeopathic prescribing. Assessment of mental and emotional state of the patient (mental symptoms) is of great importance in case taking. Therefore totality of the symptoms include not only presenting signs, concomitants, local or particular symptoms, symptoms applied to the general condition of the patient but also mental symptoms. The concept of totality is vital in homeopathy as it sets the disease in holistic frame work rather than on the named disease. Complete assessment of the patient becomes more important in chronic diseases as chronically ill patient requires succession of medicines prescribed on the basis of the changes in the patient subsequent to dosing of previous medicine. In acute diseases, matching of patient local symptoms with the homeopathic medicine may be sufficient. In case of diarrhea, information with respect to consistency and characteristics of the feces (presence of blood, mucus, or gas) aggravating or ameliorating symptoms (modalities), presence or absence of straining along with mental symptoms , is of great significance. More than one medicine may be chosen to cover all aspect of the case

Selection of Dose, Frequency and Remedy

In homeopathy, correct stimulus to regain health or cure an ailment depends not only on the selection of correct drug but also on correct potency, correct frequency and correct duration of stimulus (therapeutic duration).

Dosage in homeopathy is more related to observable dynamic of the body and the disease rather than body size i.e. it is the response of the body and disease to the drug. That's why the potency and frequency of the drug is more important. In homeopathy 'Dose' is not the number of tablet, drops, amount of powder or volume of injectable drug but it is its potency, frequency and duration of the drug. Higher potency is recommended in cases of acute disease having a prominent robust dynamic and mental symptoms. Whereas lower potency are selected for chronic disease having weaker constitutions and predominance of local pathology.

Frequency of dosing is generally chosen as per disease dynamics and the response of the animal or patient to the homeopathic drug. In acute diseases more frequent dosing at short intervals is required. While less frequent dosing (single dose or infrequent doses) is required in chronic diseases. The key to dosing of a homeopathic drug is only when the effect of first dose has worn off and symptoms persists.

The duration of the therapy is not fixed but is governed by the response of the animal/ human to the homeopathic drug. The therapy is continued only for the period necessary for regaining health i.e. as soon body responds, the drug dosing is ceased allowing the body to make use of stimulus .

The selection of Remedy in homeopathy is mainly depends on the patient's symptomology rather than the name of disease. For example a dog is not given medicine for parvo but homeopathic drug is selected on the basis of patient's reaction to illness i.e. nature and frequency of vomiting, stool, alertness or dullness, activeness or no activity, condition of the body, its mental response and desires to feed or water intake and so many associated manifestations. It means homeopathic drug may be different for different dogs suffering from the same disease. A particular drug may treat many different ailments in different animals if the symptoms manifested by the individual fits well the general picture of the homeopathic remedy. For example, homeopathic *Arsenic album* can be selected for treating gastroenteritis, peritonitis, renal disease, asthma, skin disease, nocturnal restlessness and many other conditions provided the manifestations shown by the animal/human match with the picture of *Arsenic album*.

Types of Remedies

There are various types of Homeopathic remedies such as Singular remedy, Specific remedy, Polycrest remedy, Non-polycrest remedy, Constitutional remedy and Combination remedy etc.

Singular Remedies

In homeopathy, emphasis is given on individualizing a homeopathic medicine to a sick patient i.e. on the basis of patient ailment a single medicine is chosen, Example- *Arnica* in cases of injury.

Specific Remedies

Specific remedies are nosode which are used to treat a similar infectious disease. Example- Mastitis nosode for mastitis, Cat influenza nosode for feline leucopenia.

Polycrest Remedies

- Although the method of manufacturing homeopathic remedies has changed since Hahnemann's days , his principles are still utilized today. Many reputed companies have produced over- the –counter homeopathic single and composite remedies as *Nux vomica*, *Rhus tox*, *Arsenic album* and *Calc. carb*. As these remedies are treating a wide range of common ailments they are called as polycrest remedies. In other words a remedy having many uses and used to treat many ailments is a Polycrest remedy. A polycrest remedy is a deep acting and extensively applicable remedy that affects all or nearly all tissue of the body and is useful both in acute and chronic ailments. A polycrest remedy has a potential to treat many ailments. Dr. Hahnemann has defined polycrest as " remedies in which the majority of symptoms correspond in similarity to some common disease and can therefore often be effectively applied". Polycrest remedies cover a lots of symptoms belonging to various ailments and are capable of effectively treating so many different ailments. In simple words"Polychrest" means remedies for many uses, or many ailments and used most frequently in all cases. It is to be kept in the mind that when a remedy is selected for a particular set of symptoms, the person may not necessarily have all the symptoms indicated under that medicine. There are no definite number of polycrest remedies .It varies from 25 to 90 .The homeopathic polycrest is a group of medicines which include the most symptoms to treat having a potential to restore the mental, emotional and physical health of the patient. It is mentioned that a polycrest remedy has many wide spread uses covering mental, emotional and physical symptomology as shown in proving and clinical applications.

- Well known polycrest remedies are *Aconitum, Aloe, Antimony, Apis, Agentum nitricum, Arnica montana, Arsenic album, Alumina, Baptisia, Belladonna, Bryonia, Carbo veg, Calcarea carbonica, Cantheris, Caulophyllum, Causticum, Chamomilla, Chelidonium, China, Cimicifuga, Cina, Colchicum, Colocynthis, Gelsemium, Graphite, Hamamelis, Hepar sulph, Iodum, Ipecacuanha, Kali brom., Kali carb, Lachesis, Ledum, Lycophedium, Medorrhinum, Mercuris, Natrum mur, Natrum sulph, Nitric acid, Nux vomica, Opium, Petroleum, Phosphorus, Phytolacca, Podophyllum Psorium, Pulsatila, Pyrogen, Rhus tox, Ruta, Sabina, Sepia, Silicea, Sulphur, Thuja, Veratrum, Zinc met.* etc.
- Identification of Polycrest Remedy-A polycrest remedy can be identified from sphere of action, mental emotional picture, characteristic symptoms (mental or physical), and general modalities. Many polycrest remedies have similar or identical features making it difficult to select. For example phosphorus and causticum.
- Characteristics of Polycrest Remedies- Four permeating characteristics of Polychrest remedies are Apathy, ranging from languor to torpor, Relief from rest and aggravation from motion, Sharp, stitching pains, Relief of all conditions, except the headache and eye symptoms, by warmth. Constitutional or basic Polychrest remedies are the Polycrest remedies selected mainly on the basis of the mental and physical general symptoms and to a limited extent on the basis of physical particular symptoms. Examples: *Thuja, Lachesis, Iodium, Silica, Lycopodium, Sulphur, Sepia, Petroleum, the Calcareas, the Kalis, the Natrums, Carbo vegetabilis and animalis, Graphites, Causticum, Nitric acid, Nux Vomica, Ignatia.*

Non-polycrest Remedies

- A remedy having a specific use can be called non-polycrest remedy. Actually there is no specific terminology as non-polycrest remedy. Example of speficic remedy are *Bacillinum* (for tuberculosis) , *Bora*x (for noise phobia)etc. Other non-polycrest drugs are *Aethusa cynapium, Bellis perennis, Berberis vulgaris, Cal fluorica, Cal phosphorica, Cal sulph, Calendula, Conium, Echinacea, Ferrum Phos,Hydrastis Hypericum, Ignatia amara, Kreosotum, Mag phos, Millefolium, Staphisagria, Symphyticum, Syphilinum, Urtica urens etc.*

Constitutional Remedies

- Constitutional remedies are those remedies that takes the entire constitution (make up) of the patient (sick animal, sick man) in to account rather than presenting symptom alone. The remedy matches the pattern of an individual body's programmed response to disease. These remedies have significant effect on every organ of the body.

Combination Remedies

- Despite the emphasis on individualizing a homeopathic medicine to an ailing patient by traditional homeopaths, homeopathic combination remedies- a mixture of synergistic homeo drugs for wider range are gaining popularity during recent days owing to their broad spectrum and their ability to cover many manifestations of the particular disease. Homeopathic combination remedies or complexes are the mixture of various homeopathic drugs, each medicine known to be effective for treating slightly different variations of a certain ailment. These medicines are broad spectrum remedy, which may provide benefit to a number of animals (having a little variation of an ailment). These formulations provide relief for acute nature of animal's condition, they do not usually elicit a deep curative response, as do correctly chosen single medicine (Ullman, 1998). Example- Sulphur suits the hot, dirty, thirsty, philosophical, cool seeking,, sweet loving animal that usually suffers skin disease and whose symptoms are often worse in very early morning. While Arsenic better suits the neat, fastidious individual who dislike cold, has thirst for small quantities of water, is restless, and often suffers the worst symptoms around mid night.

Destructive Remedies

- Destructive remedies are those remedy suited to syphilitic miasm. The picture of such a remedy is one of the tissue destruction.

Selection of the Remedy

Selection of homeopathic drug/remedy is based on matching of symptoms of the drug in the patient. The drug can be selected at various level.

- At a pathologic level – The remedy is selected as per disease. Example -*Arnica* is selected for injury.
- At a local level- The remedy is selected on the basis of few predominant signs and symptoms. This type of selection is valuable in acute uncomplicated disease in otherwise healthy and robust individuals. Example- *Arsenic allbum* or *Mercurius solibulus* is selected for gastroenteritis or *Colycynth* is selected for colic.
- At organotropic level- The remedy is selected on the basis of which organ is perceived to be involved. Example- *Chelidonium* is selected if liver is perceived to be involved in disease process; *Euphrasia* is selected if ailment is related to eyes; *Rhus Tox* is selected if muscle is involved; and *Symphyticum* is selected if there is bone fracture..
- At a historical level- When any particular historical incidence might have contributed greatly to the disease. Example – When trauma or injury is responsible for the disease, *Arnic*a is the choicest remedy. *Caulophyllum* is the remedy of choice when giving birth is a problem.
- Regulatory level- Homeopathic potencies of metabolites, dietary factors or poisons are selected to facilitate metabolism, absorption or excretion of a particular substance. Example- *Ferrum* is selected to aid iron absorption, *Calcarea* is selected to aid calcium metabolism. In lead toxicity where lead excretion is required, *Plumbum* is the remedy of choice.
- At a specific level- Homeopathic remedies are also selected for specific purpose to deal with infectious disease. These remedies are very specific and nosodes made from infectious material fall in this category. These remedies are used to treat similar infections. Example- Nosodes for mastitis or nosode for feline panleucopenia.
- At a desensitizing level- Homeopathic potency of allergen is used to desensitize. Example- use of homeopathic allergen in canine atopy.
- At a constitutional level- It is most important selection of the remedy based on patient's constitution. Constitutional remedies take into account the nature and individuality of the patient as a whole including his mental and physical characteristics. In selection of constitutional remedies, emphasis is given on mental symptoms as well as strange and peculiar symptoms (Hahnemann 1833-1834). Example- *Sulphur*

suits the hot, dirty, philosophical, cool seeking, sweet loving animal that suffers skin disease and whose symptoms are worst in the morning. While *Arsenic album* suits a the neat, fastidious individual who dislikes cold, has small thirsts and is restless. Symptoms in this case are worst at mid night.

Care of Homeopathic Remedies

Homeopathic remedies are delicate and required to be handled with care. Medicine taken out of the bottle should not be returned back to the bottle. Therefore required dose should only be dispensed at each dosing time. Homeopathic medicines are required to be stored away from sunlight in a cool dark place having no strong smelling substances as well as away from any electromagnetic field..

Forms of Homeopathic remedies

Homeopathic remedies are available in following forms.

- *Pillules*- Pillules are small granule like structures charged with homeopathic drug. The pills can be directly dropped in the mouth. If it is not acceptable to the patients, pills may be dissolved in small amount of boiled and cooled water in a syringe and the administered orally as liquid. For caged birds and other small exotic pets pillules may be added to drinking water freshly each day.
- *Drops*- Drops are another form in which homeopathic medicines are available. Drops can be placed directly on the tongue or added to drinking water. Cats can lick a few drops of the medicine off their nose without any stress. In birds, drops can be applied to upper beak area.
- *Powder*- Homeopathic medicines in powdered form can be poured directly in to the mouth. Not recommended for birds.
- *Injections*-This form of homeopathic drug is generally not favored by homeopaths. Many veterinarians are using this form.
- *Ointment*- This form of homeopathic drug is for external application.

Dosing Time- When more than one homeopathic medicines are to be given, the doses should be administered at different times (at least 5 to 10 minutes interval between two medicines). Homeopathic medicines should also not to be given within 15-20 minutes of feed.

References

Hahnemann,S. Organon of Medicine. Eds 5th and 6th.,New Delhi India 1833-1834. B.Jain

Mondal DTC (2006a) Health, in Spirit of the Organon. B Jain Publishers (P) Ltd, India, p. 81-84.

Mondal DTC (2006b) Disease, in Spirit of the Organon. B Jain Publishers (P) Ltd, India,pp.103-108..

Mondal DTC (2006c) Constitution, in Spirit of the Organon. B Jain Publishers (P) Ltd, India,p. 49-58.

Mondal DTC (2006d) Cure, in Spirit of the Organon. B Jain Publisher (P) Ltd, India, pp. 145-162.

Mondal DTC (2006e) Vital Force, in Spirit of the Organon. B Jain Publisher (P) Ltd, India, pp. 71-79.

Ullman,D.(1998).Homeopathic Medicine: Principles and Research.In:Complemetary and Alertnative Veterinary Medicine. Principles and Practice. Schoen, A.M. and Wynn, S.G. (1998). Mosby.

WHO (1946) Preamble to the Constitution of the World Health Organization. WHO, New York, USA

5

Analysis and Evaluation of Symptoms

Analysis of Symptoms

Symptoms are deviation from a state of health perceptible to by the patient, people around and the doctor/veterinarian. Symptoms can be physical and mental. Symptoms narrated by the patients are subjective and observed by the doctor / veterinarian are objective. Animals lack subjective symptoms. The word analysis means “careful examination of the different parts or details of something.” According to Castro “The act of resolving or reducing or breaking the whole in to pieces or groups is called analysis”. When analyzing a case, the value of symptoms is taken in to consideration on several points such as personality, and categories of symptoms as subjective, objective, general, common and uncommon symptoms. Symptom analysis gives an opportunity to learn when the symptoms developed, the feeling that those circumstances evoked the symptoms, and the ways in which those symptoms may have served some useful purpose to the patient. The main purpose of analysis is to identify the prescribing symptom in the given case.

Different Concept of Symptoms

There are different concepts of categorizing patients’ symptoms.

Hahnemann Concept - Hahnemann has classified symptoms in two categories as more striking, singular, uncommon and peculiar (characteristics) symptoms; and more general and undefined symptoms (Aphorism 153).

Kentian Concept- Kent has categorized symptoms as general, particular and common. Both symptoms and remedies are graded accordingly.

Boenninghausen’s Concept - Boenninghausen has emphasized that the individual symptoms are not important but groups are more important and patients’ symptoms are to be considered from the group aspect of location, sensation, modality, concomitants. In this method only remedies are graded and evaluated in therapeutic pocket book.

Spalding’s Method- He has classified symptoms as mental generals, physical generals, discharges, dreams, special senses, desires, aversions, modalities, strange rare and peculiar, and objective.

Dr. P. Sankaran Concept -He divided symptoms in to pathognomonic and non-pathognomonic.

Garth Boerick Concept - He divided symptoms in to basic and determinative symptoms. Basic or absolute symptoms are similar to Hahnemann's more general & undefined symptoms.

Boger's Concept- According to him, analysis is assembling of symptoms in to those of the patient and those of the disease – means Pathognomonic & non pathognomonic symptoms. The final analysis of every case therefore resolves itself in to the assembling of the individualistic symptoms in to one group and collecting the disease manifestation in to another ". (Study of MM by Boger)

Dr. N. Ghata Concept– He divided the symptoms in to Subjective & Objective categories. The subjective symptoms has been subclassified in to personal (relating to the patient as a whole) and local symptoms (relating to localities).

Most of the authors divided the symptoms in to general characteristics (rare, uncommon, peculiar, strange) and particular.

Evaluation of Symptoms

Evaluation of symptoms entails grading or ranking of different kinds of symptoms in order of priority to be matched with the symptoms of the drug. Evaluation of symptoms is a process that determines the significance and importance of expressed symptoms. Basically symptoms are ranked according to their intensity, how deeply they reach in to the organism (mental, will and emotional symptoms) and according to their degree of peculiarity. Kent has emphasized that all symptoms of will and affections including desires and aversions are the most important as they relate to the innermost of the man followed by symptoms relating to intellect. Symptoms of memory are to be ranked lowest. Elizebeth wright was of the opinion that we should not hunt in the haystack for tiny mental symptoms to open the case. The symptom should have the same importance and same weight in the patients as is assigned to them in the symptom hierarchy.

Methods of Evaluation of Symptoms

The following methods have been suggested for evaluation of symptoms.

- **Kentian method**- Kent introduced for the first time the scheme of analysis, evaluation & gradation of symptom to reach the similimum. He has given highest emphasis to mental generals reflecting the inner most of the patient.
- **Hahnemannian method**- He categorized the symptoms in to generals and uncommon.

- **Boenninghausen's method-** His emphasis was on peculiar constitution and temperament, nature of disease, seat of the disease, concomitants, cause of the disease modalities of circumstances and time of modalities.
- **Spalding-** He has classified symptoms as mental generals, physical generals, dream, special sense, desires and aversions, modalities, strange, rare peculiars, particulars, objective or pathology.
- **Whitman-** He stressed on mental general, physical general with modalities, food, desires and aversions, menses, strange rare peculiars and particulars.

Literature Consulted

Elizebeth.W. A brief study course in Homoeopathy

Hahnemann Organon of Medicine.Patel The art of case taking.

Mohanty N. "Text Book of Homoeopathic Repertory" Fourth Reprint Edition, September 2007, Indian Books & Periodical Publishers, New Delhi

Sivaraman Analysis and evaluation of symptoms.

Tiwari S.K. "Essentials of Repertorisation" Reprint edition 2006, 2007, B. Jain Publishers (P) Ltd.New Delhi.

6

Origin and Source of Homeopathic Drugs

Major source of common homeopathic drugs are plants, animals and minerals and the drug is prepared by dilution and vigorous shaking.

Origin and Source of Homeopathic Drugs

Homeopathic medicines/drugs are prepared from following sources.

Plant Source

Homeopathic drugs are prepared from different parts of the plants and herbs viz. whole plant, whole herb, flowers, stem, leaves, bark, root and seeds. Example- *Aconite, Belladonna, Arnica, Bryonia, Calendula* etc.

Animal Source

Homeopathic drugs are also prepared from some parts of animals (worms, insects, flies, lizard, crabs, toads and snakes) and their secretion. Example- *Coccus cacti, Lachesis, Naja tripudians* etc.

Mineral Source

Most of the elements and compounds like salts, metals, nonmetals, alkalis and acids are used for preparing homeopathic medicines. Example -*Sulphur, Phosphorus*, *Ferrum* etc.

Other Sources

Other sources for making another class of homeopathic drugs are infectious agents, endocrines and natural or artificial energy source. Therefore, Nosode (prepared from infectious agents), Sarcode (prepared from endocrine glands) and Imponderablilia (prepared from energy either from natural or artificial source) are the other class of homeopathic medicines. There is yet another class of homeopathic medicine called "Tautopathic "medicine, used to remove bad effects of other medications.

Nosodes - The word nosode is derived from the Greek "nosos" (disease) and "eidos" (like). Nosodes are potentized remedies prepared from diseased tissues, discharges (products of disease) or disease causing agents (bacteria or virus) in a specialized manner following standard protocol. Dr. Samuel

Hahnemann first prepared remedies from diseased tissues (mainly the miasmatic nosodes) for the three miasms (Psora, Sycosis and Syphilis) correspondingly known as Psorinum, Medorrhinum, and Syphylinum. Of which first two have common use in veterinary homeopathy. The nosodes underwent provings similar to other drugs, and their use in veterinary homeopathy is the same as with any other remedy i.e. matching patient symptoms with those of the remedy. Later in the 1800s, the use of nosodes developed for specific diseases, started such as anthrax in cattle (Anthracinum), and distemper in dogs (Distemperinum).Later on a nosode Hydrophobinum (30c potency) was developed from the saliva of the rabid dog by Dr. Constantine Hering to treat and prevent rabies in dogs and humans. Now a days this nosode is known as "Lyssin". Heart worm and Parvo nosodes also offer some promise to boost immunity .These medicines are not antibiotics and do not possess bactericidal or bacteriostatic activity (Banerjee, 2006). Examples of nosodes used in humans are Baccilinum (from tuberculous sputum), medorrhinum (from gonorrhea agent), carcinosin (from cancerous tissues); psorinum (psoric preparation), pyrogenium (infected pus), syphilinum (syphilitic germs' preparation), tuberculinum (pus of tubercular abscess), typhoidinum (*Salmonella typhi*' preparation), variolinum (smallpox eruptions' preparation), Ambra grisea (whale), aviare (tuberculin vof chicken), anthracinum (anthrax poison from spleen of affected cattle or sheep), mallandrinum (grease in horse), hydrophobinum or lyssin (saliva of a rabid dog), Secale cor (fungus growing on the seeds of the secale cerale), and ustilago maydis (fungus, growing on the stem of Indian corn).The recorded use of nosode in animals dates back to 1831 when Wilhelm Lux used 30CH dilution of a drop of mucus from glander affected animal (AAHP and AHVMA,1991). Nosodes have also been used in Livestock (Day, 1995, Macleod, 1981,1991. 1994). Nosodes have been tried for kennel cough, distemper, hepatitis and parvo in dogs, for influenza, enteritis, feline leukemia virus and feline infectious peritonitis in cats; and influenza and herpes in horses (Day, 1998).

Sarcodes- Sarcodes are prepared from endocrine glands (adrenaline, pancreas, pituitary, thyroid, ovaries or testicle) and their secretions. Examples of sarcode are *Adrenalinum* (secretion produced by adrenal glands), *pancreatinum* (pancreas of beef animals), *insulin* (pancreatic hormones), pituitary (posterior portion of the pituitary gland of sheep), pepsinum (digestive enzyme pepsin), cholesterinum, thyroidinum (thyroid gland) , oophorinum (ovary of cow or sheep), orchitinum (testicular), etc.

Imponderablilia - These are the medicines made from energy, either from natural or artificial source (Wadhwani, 2011). Even many imponderable (immaterial) substances can produce most violent medicinal effects on human beings. The medicines from this source include: Luna (full moon), magnetis polus Australia (South Pole of the magnet), magnetis polus Arcticus (North Pole of magnet), magnetis poli ambo (magnet), sol (sun rays), radium, Magnetis artificialis, electricitus, and X-ray (Banerjee, 2006). Hahnemann writes, "Even many imponderable (immaterial) substances can produce most violent medicinal effects on human beings". (Organon, aphorisms 280).

References and Literature reviewed

American Association of Homeopathic Pharmacists and the American Holistic Veterinary Medical Association. (1991). The place of homeopathic remedies in veterinary medicine., 1991,

Banerjee, D.(2006). Augmented Textbook of Homoeopathic Pharmacy: B. Jain Publishers (P) Ltd,

Day, C. (1995). Homeopathic treatment of beef and dairy cattle, Beaconsfield, England, Beaconsfield Publisher.

Day, C. (1998). Veterinary Homeopathy: Principles and Practice. In: Complementary and Alternative Veterinary Medicine. Principles and Practice. Schoen, A.M. and Wynn, S.G. (eds). Mosby, St Louis, baltomore, Boston,Carlsbad, Chicago, Naples, New York, Philadelphia, Portland, London, Madrid, Mexico City, Sigapore, Sydney, Tokyo, Toronto, Wiesbaden.pp 485-513.

Macleod,G. (1981). Treatment of cattle by homeopathy.Saffron Walden, England. CW Daniel

Macleod,G. (1991). Goats:homeopathic remedies..Saffron Walden, England. CW Daniel.

Macleod,G. (1994). A Veterinary Materia Medica.Saffron Walden, England. CW Daniel.

Wadhwani G.G. (2011). Imponderabilia in Homeopathic Practice.Amer. J. Hom. Med. 104:131.

7

Homeopathic Prescribing in Animals

Many human illnesses are contacted from animals and plants; and are also due to imbalance in the environment. Mental, emotional and relational symptoms seen in humans are absent in animals. Nevertheless, careful observations on the behavior of the animal and its relation with others may play key role in homeopathic prescribing in animals. No doubt the use of homeopathy in animals is challenging. Homeopathic treatment of pet animals has many similarities with homeopathic treatment of babies and children such as non-verbal communication, the socialization and the relationship with third parties (owners in case of pets and parents in case of children).There are many prescribing strategies in veterinary homeopathy.

Types of Homeopathy Practice in Animals

Homeopathy in animals is being practiced as an exclusive or sole homeopathic practice, second opinion homeopathic practice or as referral homeopathic practice broadly in a manner similar to humans. In India homeopathic practice in animals is being done casually as an adjunct with modern drugs by mostly unqualified practitioners. There are neither separate homeopathic clinics for animals nor separate veterinarian trained in homeopathy. But for full benefit of homeopathy, species variations demand specific approach in homeopathic prescribing for an individual animal.

History in Animals

History in animals, a very important component for homeopathic prescribing, is entirely depended on the observational power of the owner because of non-verbal nature of expression in animals. A correct detailed history in free ranging or grazing animals (sheep and goat) is a difficult task to obtain as animal contact with their keepers is minimal. History of subtle symptoms (an essential in the field of homeopathy) is mostly absent in animals as quality of sensation in pain is not appreciable in animals. Modalities are also dependent on objective observations. Careful history-taking and observation along with knowledge of normal behavior of the species and individual is required to make an appropriate distinction. A veterinary repertory undoubtedly offers some help in selecting rubrics for animals.

Mental and Emotional Symptoms in Animals

Animals are incapable of providing a single direct mental symptoms. At best interpretations can be derived from animal behavior in terms of human emotions. Close observations in animals may provide useful information to attending veterinary homeopath. But emotions being experienced by the animal cannot be ascertained. Human homeopaths gives more emphasis on mental and emotional symptoms in case analysis. It is rather impractical in case analysis in animals for veterinary prescribing. Veterinarian has to face problems (unique to animals) in relation to obstacles to cure. Management and feeding regimes frequently create a situation in which homeopathic drug has to struggle to act with any consistency.

Veterinary Patients

For the sake of convenience veterinary patients can be categorized as pet animals (dog, cats, small furry animals and small reptiles), performance animals (horses, racing greyhound dogs and working sheep dogs), food producing animals (cloven footed animals, poultry) and wild and exotic animals (zoo animals, leporine, exotic birds etc.).

In urban areas most of the veterinary practices devote to the treatment of companion animals having much strong human-animal bond and owner concern for their welfare because of intense emotions. As canine and feline diseases are in many ways similar to that of humans, their homeopathic treatment is extrapolated from the human models closely. Companion animal clinics are flooded with the cases of chronic ailments such as osteo-arthritis, aural hematoma, urinary incontinence, ataxia, paralysis, jaundice, chronic hepatic disease, chronic renal disease, chronic skin disease, colitis and associated bowel disorders, chronic respiratory disease and behavioral problems etc. Many of cases comes as referral after much desperation.

In performance animals, homeopathy can assist in maintaining their peak fitness and redressing their injuries. Epistaxis due to over exertion in racing thoroughbred horses can not only be treated but also its propensity can be reduced by homeopathic drug *Vipera*. Another important area is chronic fatigue syndrome in race horses that can be effectively addressed by homeopathy. The horse as a species seems to be extremely sensitive to homeopathy. It is considered that 30c potencies do well in horses.

Homeopathy is being increasingly practiced in producing animals under organic farming throughout the world by Veterinarians as well as farmers themselves. Practice of homeopathy in food producing animals is most challenging as the concept of individualization is least relevant as an animal is seen more as an economic unit and a large number of animals in the herd or a flock make it practically difficult to individualize every animal for treatment. This has necessitated the development of strategies for prescribing for the groups.

Homeopathy also holds promise in wild animals whether rescued after injury, captured or transported. Shock and bruising in rescued wild animals can be readily and effectively treated with homeopathy. Liquid homeopathic remedies can be dropped onto the nose of the rescued animal or by the use of aqueous spray or water supply in dangerous unmanageable animals. These means of drug administration can overcome the problem of drug administration in wild animals.

Prescribing Homeopathy in Veterinary Practice

There are different grounds (causation to pathogen) on which the practice of homeopathy is done in animals.

i. *Causation* -At present in India the prescribing of homeopathic drugs in veterinary field is mostly based on Causation using first aid homeopathic remedies. *Arnica* and *Hypericum* is generally prescribed in cases of skin abrasions/lacerations as well as road traffic injuries. These cases are viewed in the pathogenic model as their histories clearly reflect trauma as etiology. Grief in animals specially dogs is most commonly identified mental causality owing to their close relationship with their owners, offsprings, mother or other species (when interspecies friendship develops). Loss of any close companion may put them in the state of grief corresponding to the remedy picture of *Ignatia* or *Natrum mur*. Even rehoming may put them in the state of grief. The situation can also be dealt with prescribing of *Ignatia* or *Natrum mur*. It has been reported that the cat belonging to an owner (who has just suffered from bereavement), may pick up on owner's emotions and symptoms corresponding to the *Natrum mur* .

   The specific reaction to grief may be different in different circumstances. A calm and compose dog may sometimes apparently become aggressive in the event of loss of head of the family. Such aggrieved dogs with arthritis and hind limb weakness may respond well to *Causticum* (identifiable from etiology alone).

   Homeopaths think the animal vaccination, though has controlled many serious diseases, is causing a cost to the general health of the animal population as a whole because vaccinations tend to cause or worsen chronic disease. This is a debatable issue. Atopic dermatitis, colitis and epilepsy seem to be exacerbated by vaccination. Any such situation appearing within three months of vaccination is being considered to be suspicious; within one month even more so. Majority of such cases would respond to *Thuja occidentalis*.

ii. *Local Prescribing*- The difficulty of getting complete history from animals can be overcome by prescribing based on directly observable symptoms (objective symptoms) and signs of the disease and a full examination of the ailing animal. In many aged ailing animals clinical manifestations are exhibited lately only when much pathology has progressed and set in; and mental symptoms are obscured, local prescribing seems appropriate. When local symptom is strange, rare or peculiar, it gives more support to local prescribing. Concomitant symptoms, modalities and characteristic symptoms are very important in homeopathic case analysis. Involvement of owner in the process of making diagnosis and prescribing may be very fruitful. His minute feelings and observations can often be validated and are important in veterinary homeopathy. In case of canine diarrhea, owner's information regarding consistency and color of the feces, frequency and time, and dog's reaction on scolding is valuable in finding appropriate homeopathic remedy.

iii. *Holistic Approach (with mental signs*)- Interpretation of mental and emotional states in animals is a little problematic. It is more in rodents, reptiles and terrapins. Careful detailed observations of the behavior of the ailing animal and narration of the sensitive owner may provide some leads with respect to emotional state of the animal. The interpretation of the behavior of the animal is influenced by emotional state of the owner as well as of veterinarian to some extent. For example fear reaction of dog to thunder may be due to noise phobia or due to atmospheric changes. Accurate interpretation of mental states requires sound knowledge of behavior of the species.

iv. *Constitution and Breed*- In chronic diseases with clear cut symptoms, prescribing may be on constitutional lines. An assessment of general physical attribute of the ailing animal may help in constitutional prescription. To cite an example, A flat, chilly Labra with swollen joint reluctant to exercise will probably respond to *Calcarea carbonica*. In chronic diseases, constitutional remedy will yield desirable results. Heredity hip dysplasia is more common in some breeds such as German Shepherds. In homeopathy it can be taken as breed tendency to show features of specific constitution. Golden Labrador's exhibit features of *Calcarea carbonica* constitution.

v. *Multiple Prescribing*- Many veterinarians, practicing homeopathy, prefer to give more than one remedy as 'gold standard' of prescribing single medicine based on the totality of symptoms and constitution needs a fairly long period of observation before the drug is repeated. Multiple drug prescribing covers aspects of totality or different local symptoms. Nowadays many commercial homeopathic mixtures containing more than one homeopathic drugs are available for specific disease indication. These combination remedies are effective in treating the local symptoms.

vi. *Obstacles Removal for Cure*- Many animals refractory to undergoing modern treatment are referred for homeopathic treatment. Such cases have suppressed symptom and need clearing remedies (*Sulphu*r or *Nux vomica*) first before prescribing classical homeopathic remedies. The purpose of clearing remedies is to remove the obstacles for cure and to create clear clinical picture. Another obstacle to recovery is continued feeding of processed commercial dry and pelleted food. A healthy diet should have healthy ingredient preferably organic and should be free from harmful additives, be fresh and minimally processed or not processed at all. Convenient diets containing additives should be avoided as far as possible .From homeopaths point of view, a diet on natural plane is more desirable and appropriate. Drinking water should also be of good quality. Plastic or aluminum feed containers, bowels, mangers or cooking utensils should be avoided. Animals should normaly be given adequate exercise. In close animal spaces, human smoking should be prohibited.

vii. *Prescribing for groups of Animals* – Animals kept in group (be it dogs in kennels, milking cows in herd or poultry in flock) create difficulty in individualization. Problems in the group of animals may be infectious (viral, bacterial, protozoal, rickettsial or fungal), non-infectious or food related (deficiency or toxicity). A uniform response from a group of animals may be produced. Based on predominant symptoms, a single remedy (similar to symptoms based on simillinium philosophy) can be selected and can be given to all affected ones in the group. Example- *Thuja* for orf. *Caulophyllu*m has been proved effective in preventing stillbirths in sow (Day,1984). *Sepia* has been found effective in improving calving–to-service interval in dairy herd (Williamson *et al.*,1995). In metabolic and deficiency diseases, appropriate mineral in homeopathic potency may be rewarding. In outbreaks, symptomology may vary considerably in the group and there may be 3 or 4 distinct symptoms indicating different remedies. In such cases these remedies may be mixed and given to the whole group.

viii. *Prescribing of Nosodes* - The use of nosodes is based on the involvement of specific pathogen (microbial etiological agent). The use of nosodes is called as isopathy as it is based on the specific pathogen rather than symptoms. Nosodes have been used in the control of mastitis in cows (Day, 1986).

Administration Methods

- Tablets or pillules are swallowed in humans. This way of administration of homeopathic drugs in true sense is not feasible in animals. It is better to administer homeopathic drugs as liquid or powder in animals. Liquid remedies in the form of drops or spray can be directly applied to oral or nasal mucus membranes. Occasionally homeopathic drugs can be given to dogs mixed with bland foods (bread). Oral dosing of homeopathic drugs to large animals is a little problematic. The liquid medicines can be sprayed into the vulva in cows or onto the muzzle of sheep and goats. Injectable form of the remedies may also be used if feasible. The most common method of administration of homeopathic drugs to large animals is mixing the remedy in drinking water of the individual animal. Ointments can be applied locally.

Repetition of Homeopathic Drugs

- Animals may require more frequent and more prolonged drug administration.
- Initial Course of homeopathy in an animal can consists of 30 c potency given daily for a week. When given as add on with conventional therapy, it may be given continuously for some weeks.

References

Day, C. (1984).Control of stillbirths using homoeopathy.Vet Rec 114:216

Day, C.(1986). Clinical trials in bovine mastitis using nosodes for prevention. Int. J. Vet. Hom.1:15

Day, C.(1995). The homoeopathic treatment of beef and dairy cattle. Beaconsfield Publishers, Beaconsfield, UK.

Williamson, A. V., Mackie, W. L., Crawford, W. J. and Rennie, B.(1995). A trial of Sepia 200: prevention of anoestrus problems in dairy cows. Br Homoeopathic J 84(1):14–20

Literature Reviewed

Day, C .(1998). The homeopathic treatment of small animals, 3rd edn. C W Daniel, Saffron Walden.

Gregory, P. (2007). Veterinary Prescribing. In: Principles and Practices of Homeopathy. Owen, D.(editor). Churchill Livingstone Elsevier. pp237-250.

Hamilton, D. (1999).Homeopathic care for cats and dogs. North Atlantic Books, Berkeley.

8

Homeopathic Prescription and Posology

Homeopathic Prescription

A basis for homeopathic prescription involves identifying all the aspects of the case (detailed questioning to get the history in respect to animal, its behavior, its nutrition and management, vaccination and deworming status, past and present illness etc.), objective investigations (instrumental and laboratory), coupled with an overview of the picture and dynamics of the patient (it is more philosophical and subjective).

In recording symptoms (both present and past), special attention is to be paid to peculiar symptoms, mental state and generalities. Then appropriate remedy is selected through a process called "reportization". After selecting an appropriate remedy, its correct potency is determined. Selection of the potency depends on the strength of vital force of the ailing individual, degree and extent of physical pathology and disease chronicity (Hahnemann,1994). Higher potency is selected if vital force is strong. For example higher potency are more suitable for young and growing animals. If tissue pathology is more, lower potency drug is advisable. The effect of higher potency drugs is for greater period of time. Effect of 1M potency may last for a month while that of 30C potency may last for a week. If pathology is not severe, 200C potency may be selected. In case pathology is significant, potency below 200C may be chosen. For weak and emaciated animals, potency 30C or below is advisable. Clear cut cases with strong mental symptoms are right candidates for high potency. Unclear case should be given low potency drug (Pitcairn, 1992). As soon as relief is observed, the drug administration should be stopped. Overmedication is the great error in homeopathic prescribing. In homeopathic prescribing, number of pillules taken in a single dose is less important. What matters is its potency and frequency.

Homeopathic drugs should be avoided with strong aromatic products as well as concomitant use of allopathic medicines. Homeopathic drugs should not be touched with hand and should be kept away from sun light and electromagnetic radiation

Posology

The word posology has originated from the Greek word, '*posos*' and 'logos' meaning how much and study or discourse respectively. In broader sense 'Posology 'is the doctrine of doses of medicine.

Dose

The word *'dose'* has been derived from the word 'dosis' that means the quantity of a drug to be taken or applied all at a time or in fractional amounts within a stated period.

Homeopathic Posology

Homeopathic posology deals with the dose of homeopathic drug. In homoeopathy 'dose' means the particular preparation of medicine used, its quantity and form as well as frequency of administration in stipulated time. In short, homoeopathic 'dose' includes potency, quantity, form and frequency of drug administration.

In allopathy, dose relates to quantity or volume of the drug, route of administration and frequency of drug administration. While in homeopathy dose of anything means an infinitesimal dose. It relates to particular preparation of the medicine used (potency), quantity and form of that preparation, repetition (frequency of administration in a set period of time).

Fundamentals of Homeopathic Posology

Fundamentals of homeopathic posology are single remedy, minimum dose and minimum repetition.

- In the treatment of diseases, only one simple medicinal substance should be used at a time. (Aphor. 72). A simple medicinal substance when used in diseases, the totality of whose symptoms is accurately known, renders efficient aid by itself alone, if it be homeopathically selected. (Aphor. 274).
- In homoeopathy uses of minute dose has certain advantage. Well selected medicine in minute dose is sufficient to overcome and extinguish the disease and unwanted aggravation can be avoided. Minute doses are appropriate for gentle remedial effect. The specific dynamic action is produced by the minimum quantity of the drug. The smallness of the dose (minute amount of drug) does not allow the drug to do any organic damage nor there are any medium doses paralyse and large doses kill' risk of 'drug addiction and drug-effects. In order to maintain the similarity of the sequence of the disease and the drug, minimum dose

is suitable. The concept of minimum dose is verified by Arndt-Schultz law-'Small doses stimulate, medium dose paralyze and large does kill'

- Dose is repeated only when improvement ceases.

Potency Selection

Selection of potency is next to selection of drug and it is utmost important as the selected drug on the basis of totality of symptoms may not act curatively unless given in proper potency. Broadly there are three categories of homeopathic potency such as low potency (below 30c), medium potency (30c, 200c and 1M) and high potency (above 1M). It has been stated that low potencies are organotropic, medium potencies influence function, and high potencies relates to psyche. Low potencies are selected in organic disease, medium potencies are selected for functional disorders and high potencies are selected for mental symptoms.

Factors Responsible for Potency Selection

- Patient's susceptibility- more the susceptibility, less medicinal quantity and higher potency is a general rule. Susceptibility is modified by age, constitution and temperament, habit and environment, and pathological condition.

  a) Susceptiblity tends to be maximum in young ones but decreases continuously with age at a slower pace till youth and then at increasing pace till death. Therefore, medium or high potency may be chosen in young ones.

  b) Constitution and temperament also modify susceptibility. Higher potencies are best adapted to sensitive persons of the nervous, sanguine or choleric temperament, intelligent, zealous and impulsive persons. Lower potencies (large and frequent doses) correspond better to torpid and phlegmatic individuals slow to act, sluggish individuals or those with great muscular power. Medium potencies are best adapted to oversensitive patients.

  c) Habit and environment also modify susceptibility. Higher potencies are best adapted to persons in intellectual occupation, sedentary occupation, people with excitement of imagination and emotions, persons sleeping more, Lower potencies are best adapted to people accustomed to severe outdoor labour, sleeping less, eating coarse food, connected to tobacco or liquor trade, druggists, perfumers, chemical workers, idiot, deaf and dumb.

  d) Pathological conditions influence susceptibility. In certain terminal conditions, due to the existence of gross pathological lesions or of long existent, exhausting chronic disease, massive dose of crude medicine is to be administered.

- Nature and intensity of the disease- It plays significant role in potency selection. Functional diseases respond to high potencies and organic diseases to low potencies. Medium or low potencies are given in acute crisis on chronic trouble. In chronic diseases with no organic change 200 c potency is chosen. While chronic diseases with organic change responds well to lower potencies. In mental diseases, higher potency drugs are chosen.
- Stage and duration of the disease- Lower and medium potency drugs are better in incurable chronic diseases. Very high potency drugs are more appropriate in terminal stage of chronic diseases.

Kinds of Doses

- Maximum dose- It is largest amount of drug taken at a time with out any harm.
- Lethal or fatal dose- An amount of dose causing death is the lethal dose.
- Booster dose- A subsequent dose given to enhance the action of initial dose is called as booster dose.
- Fractional dose- It is the fraction of a full dose to be taken at short intervals.
- Physiological dose- It is the dose which stimulates physiology or functions of different organs.
- Minimum dose- It is the dose that is sufficient to overpower and annihilate the disease and capable of producing slight homoeopathic aggravation scarcely observable after its ingestion (Aphor. 280).It is the smallest amount of the medicine produces the least possible excitation of the vital force, and yet sufficient, to effect the necessary changes in it. (Aphor 246).

Repetition of Doses

General rules for repetition of doses are:

- As soon as an adequate response is observed, dose is not repeated.
- As long as the response continues, the drug is not repeated.
- Cessation of progress is not to be taken as an indication for repetition.
- The dose is repeated only when the symptoms return that have disappeared under the action of the remedy.

Hahnemann's instructions of repetition of doses as per the 5th edition of Organon

- It depends on the condition and progress of the patient, nature of the disease and nature of the remedy.
- Perceptible and continued progress of improvement contraindicates repetition (Aphor. 245). Dose is repeated only when improvement ceases. Repetition may be continued till either recovery ensues or different groups of symptoms arise and thus demands different remedy (Aphor. 248). The dose of the same medicine' may be repeated several times, if necessary, until recovery ensues, or until the same medicine ceases to do well.
- Repetition in new method (246 & 248 6th edition Organon) -To prevent the undesirable reactions of the vital energy, Hahnemann, after many experiment wholly solved the difficulties by giving "new altered but perfected method". In chronic disease- the same carefully selected medicine may now be given daily and for months, the lower degree of potency is used for one or two weeks, followed by higher degrees in the same way. 5. §248 6th edition-In acute diseases- every two to six hours. 6. §248 6th edition -In very urgent cases- every hour or oftener.

Kent's instructions of repetition of doses

- The first medicine should be repeated when improvement remains standstill.
- When original symptoms return after a temporary disappearance having the same general and particulars as formerly (Kent's 11th observation).

Homeopathic Dosages Forms

Homeopathic drugs are available in the following forms.

- Capsules
- Liquid for oral or sublingual administration
- Liquids and semi-solids for oro-mucosal administration
- Medicated globules
- Medicated powders
- Medicated tablets
- Nasal solutions
- Ophthalmic solutions
- Otic solutions

- Suppositories
- Topical dosage forms as ointment, gel or cream

Route of Administration of Homeopathic drugs

Homoeopathic drugs or medicines can be administered through various routes for a curative effect, such as oral route, olfaction (inhalation through nose or mouth), skin application, application of medicine through milk of mother or wet nurse, etc. Among these, the oral route is commonly preferred . Other route of drug administration can also be employed as per the requirement of case. Dr. Hahnemann has emphasized the importance of each of these modes in his Organon of Medicine. Homeopathic medicines are commonly dispensed in the form of liquid, medicated globules (containing active ingredient in a base of lactose), topical products, powder or tablets. The drugs are also available in the form of syrups, lozenges, eye drops, medicated powders, capsules containing powder or pellets, and suppositories. Alcohol is an excellent preservative and is used as vehicle for homeopathic medicines (1) Dr. Hahnemann described about the alternate modes of drug administration of homoeopathic medicines in §284 of 6th edition of Organon of Medicine as "Besides the tongue, mouth and stomach, which are most commonly affected by the administration of medicine, the nose and respiratory organs are receptive of the action of medicines in fluid form by means of olfaction and inhalation through the mouth."

Oral Route of Administration (ingestion through mouth)- The medicines, taken orally, act effectively and promptly. Potentized homeopathic medicines require no digestion. They get absorbed directly from the mouth and then act through the cerebrospinal or ganglionic nervous system (3).Homeopathic medicines taken after dissolving in water enhances its effect as the drug comes in contact with a much larger surface of sensitive nerves. Touching of homeopathic globules or tablets should be avoided. The globules or tablets should be gently placed in the mouth.

Any oils on the skin may stick on the surface of the pellets or tablets and may impede the proper absorption of the drug. For better buccal absorption, it is generally suggested that homeopathic medicines be taken with a clean mouth, away from strong flavors (e.g., strong mint or menthol products).

Sublingual administration – It is adopted in cases of coated tongue which interferes with the absorption and action of medicines. Homeopathic drugs should not be chewed . Hahnemann states about the oral mode of administration of homoeopathic medicines in § 272 of 6th edition of Organon of Medicine 6 that: "Such a globule,1 placed dry upon the tongue, is one of the smallest doses for a moderate recent case of illness. Here but few nerves are touched by the medicine. A similar globule, crushed with some sugar of milk and dissolved in a good deal of water (§247) and stirred well before every administration will produce a far more powerful medicine for the use of several days. Every dose, no matter how minute, touches, on the contrary, many nerves." These globules (§270) retain their medicinal virtue for many years, if protected against sunlight and heat.

Olfaction – It is inhalation through nose or mouth. It means 'Act of Smelling'. It is a method of administering medicine to a patient through the nose and mouth by the act of smelling. Hahnemann was administering medicines by oral routes for many years. But in his last years (1833) he favored the olfactory route. He states in the footnote of §288 of 5th edition of Organon of Medicine that 'homoeopathic remedies act most surely and most powerfully when the medicinal aura that is always emanating from the medicine is inhaled for a short time' (2).

Application to the skin-Topical products are applied directly to the skin to stimulate a localized healing process(1). These include glycerol, ointments, liniments, opodeldoc (liniment), lotions, cerates, poultices, fomentations, plasters, sprays and oils etc. The administration of the medicines through the skin is done by rubbing or enepidermic (drug is simply kept in contact with the unbroken skin without rubbing. For example as plaster, poultices, ointment).

Application of medicine through milk of mother or wet nurse- For treating ailing infants and neonates, homeopathic drugs can be given through nursing mothers. The medicines can be utilized by the child or neonate animal through the milk of the mother. About this, Hahnemann writes in the footnote of §284 of 6th edition of Organon of Medicine6 that: "The power of medicines acting upon the infant through the milk of the mother or wet nurse is wonderfully helpful. Every disease in a child yields to the rightly chosen homoeopathic medicines given in moderate doses to the nursing mother and so administered, is more easily and certainly utilized by these new world-citizens than is possible in later years."

General Instructions Regarding Administration of Homeopathic drug and Their Storage

Homeopathic medicines should be given into a clean mouth. Preferably no food should be given within 30 minutes of the drug administration. Homeopathic drugs should be stored away from sun light, away from any electromagnetic field and away from strong smell. It is advisable to store homeopathic drugs in a cupboard. Discolored medicine should be discarded.

References and Literature Reviewed

Bradford, T.L.(2016). The Life and Letter of Dr. Samuel Hahnemann. New Delhi. B.Jain Publishers Pvt Ltd. 2016

Close Stuart, (2009). The Genius Of Homoeopathy Lecture And Essay On Homoeopathic Philosophy. New Delhi. B.Jain Publishers Pvt. Ltd. 2009.

Dudgeon, R.E. (2015). Lectures on the Theory and Practice of Homoeopathy. New Delhi. B. Jain Publishers Pvt .Ltd. 2015

Dunham,C.(2015). Homoeopathy the Science of Therapeutics. New Delhi. B. Jain Publishers Pvt Ltd. 2015. 3

Hahnemann, S. (1994).Organon ofmedicine. (edited from 5th and 6th editions), Haifa, Homeopress.

Hahnemann, S. (2010). Organon of Medicine, 5th ed. New Delhi. B.Jain Publishers Pvt Ltd. 2010. 4 .

Hahnemann, S. (2013).His Life and Work, vol-1. New Delhi. B.Jain Publishers Pvt. Ltd.2013.

Hahnemann, S. (2010). Organon of Medicine, 6th ed. New Delhi. B.Jain Publishers Pvt Ltd. 2010. 4 .

Kent, J.T. (2011). Lectures on Homoeopathic Philosophy, 5th ed. New Delhi. B.Jain Publishers Pvt Ltd. 2011.

Pitcairn, R.(1992). Course notes in Certification Course for Veterinary Homeopathy, Eugene, Ore.

1.Frequently asked questions (Internet). (cited 2022 May 17). Available from: https://www.theaahp.org/consumer-information/faqs/

2.Hahnemann S. Organon of Medicine [R.E. Dudgeon, W. Boericke, trans]. 5th and 6th New Delhi: Indian Books & Periodicals Publishers; April 2004

3.Mandal PP, Mandal B. A textbook of homoeopathic pharmacy. Calcutta: New Central Book Agency (P) Ltd.; 2002

9

Case Taking in Homeopathy

Case taking in homeopathy is based on five themes such as Philosophy of Homeopathy, Materia Medica of Homeopathy, The case, Case Analysis and Case Management (Owen, 2007).

Themes

i. ***Philosophy*** – Clinical practice of homeopathy is based on the principles and key concepts of homeopathy as detailed in Chapter 2 and 12.

ii. ***Materia Medica***- It is in the core of understanding of the practice of homeopathy providing the information how the remedy pictures are developed and expressed in different ways. It allows the practitioner to understand the patient and prescribe rationally.

iii. ***The Case***- The relationship between a homeopath (human /veterinary) and patient (animal or human) is in the center of the therapeutic process in case taking in homeopathy. It is more than a record of the consultation as case skills facilitate the level of revealing by the patient and the depth to which the homeopath perceives.

iv. ***Case Analysis***- Case analysis allows the matching of what is perceived of the patient with what is known of the remedies. Case analysis governs the order, pattern and interpretation that emerge in the healing process. The variety of case analysis strategies and methodologies available to the homeopath is a major factor that determines the breadth of their clinical competence.

v. ***Case Management***- The prescribing of a homeopathic remedy is only one part of the therapeutic and healing process. Each case requires the consideration of its illness, the patient and the homeopath. In homeopathic case management, the science of the homeopathic healing, caring skill and mannerism, and the attending clinician are brought together. Homeopathic case management focusses on the process of cure and care of the patient.

Case Analysis

Case history is most important in case analysis and it should be taken as detailed as possible. For case history, an interview with the person caring the animal, should be scheduled and after that the ailing animal should be observed closely. Though the animal has feelings, motivation, desires, needs and mental stress in same way as humans, the main difference is mental. Animals have hardly any concept of future and its concomitant anxieties, stresses or hopes. Other difference is that the animals have objective symptoms only. They do not have subjective symptoms as humans have. Case study or case taking in homeopathy should consider physical signs (objective symptoms), owners complaint as well as mental considerations of the animal. In homeopathic prescribing for animals, stress is given to identify the essential nature or clinical picture being presented by the ailing animal to match with a homeopathic remedy. Therefore, general picture is more important than the conventional name of the disease. For example Parvo is not important from homeopathic point of view but clinical manifestation such as vomiting and its frequency, color, volume, and nature; nature of feces and its frequency, characteristics; desire for water; preferring cold or hot; or mental expression (dullness, dizziness, sleepiness or activeness) is more valuable to match with the homeopathic remedy. It does not emphasize to ignore the conventional diagnosis.

Identifying the detail symptomatic expression of the ailing animal to form a base for homeopathic prescribing involves not only detailed questioning but also physical examination supported by results of diagnostic tools (X-ray, ultrasound, electrocardiogram, echocardiogram etc.) and laboratory investigations. Obstacles to recovery such as poor diet, environmental stressors, lack of exercise, or saddling and shoeing in case of horses should also be addressed as these factors may inhibit the animal's response to treatment and its ability to heal .

In his Organon (1833-34), the father of homeopathy wrote the following about the qualities of a true practitioner of the healer art.

- If he (physician/veterinarian) perceives that which is to be cured in the disease.
- If he perceives what is curative in the medicine.
- If he knows how to match what is curative in medicines to what he has discovered to be wrong in the patient.
- If he knows how to adjust the potency, the frequency and the duration of the medicine.
- If he knows how to identify and to remove the obstacles to recovery.

In short, a homeopathic healer should compose a detailed, careful and emphatic case study; match the disease picture with the remedy picture and remove obstacles or adverse factors hindering the healing process.

Components of Case Analysis

- The Case study
- Selection of appropriate matching remedy
- Identifying obstacles to recovery and their removal
- Dosages
- Administration and care of homeopathic remedies
- Preventive Medicine

The Case study

- Gathering a thorough knowledge of the patient from the owner or attendant caring the ill animal. One has to be patient listener without interrupting the owner or caretaker of the animal when he is talking.
- Avoid leading questions, whose answers may distort the picture.
- The first essential part of case study is introduction to the patient. It involves observing the behavior right from the first appearance to consulting room.
- The second essential part of case study is the nature of the complaint. It not only includes presenting complaint but also includes characteristics of each symptom (if there is any discharge, its details such as color, with mucus, or pus), modalities (factors such as weather, temperature, eating, drinking and moving influencing the symptoms for good or bad), what periodicity symptoms follow i.e. when disease is worse (winter/ summer, morning/evening/ night), period of symptoms persistence, happening at the outset (ill since vaccination, injury, surgery or any change) and any problems occurring at the same time.
- The third essential part of the case study is the patient itself . It involves patient medical history, family history, mental symptoms /behavior (is the patient shy, aggressive, friendly, impulsive or steady. Reaction of the animal to music, fuss, noise or situations), general symptoms (build, physique, posture, movement, desires, aversion, thirst and response to weather, seasons etc.), particular symptom (particular or local symptom) and strange symptom (peculiar symptoms seen only in the case).
- The fourth essential part of the case study is life style, nutrition and management. It covers management and nutritional aspect of the animal.

- Cats differs in some points as far as examination process is concerned. Cats behavior under restrain in the basket as well as on the examination table, and reaction to various stimuli should be observed.
- Caged birds should be observed closely without causing too much shock, fear or any physical stress/trauma.
- In farm animals, the history may not be complete. Nevertheless, the food producing animals should be examined carefully and thoroughly. The principles of treatment of farm animals are the same as for dogs and cats or any other species. In large animals, history relating to hygiene, housing, feeding, grassland management, silage/ hay making, dietary composition and supplementation and health care procedures should always be considered.
- Other components of case study have been described in other chapters.

References and Literature Reviewed

Day, C. (1998). Veterinary Homeopathy: Principles and Practice. In : Complementary and Alternative Veterinary Medicine. Principles and Practice. Schoen, A.M. and Wynn, S.G. (eds). Mosby, St Louis, baltomore, Boston,Carlsbad, Chicago,Naples, New York, Philadelphia, Portland, London, Madrid, Mexico City, Sigapore, Sydney,Tokyo, Toronto, Wiesbaden.pp 485-513.

Owen, D. (2007). Principles and Practice of Homeopathy. The therapeutic and HealingProcess. Churchil Livingstone Elsevier.

10

Materia Medica, Pharmacy and Pharmacopeia

Materia Medica

The word 'Materia medica' is a Latin term that means medical matters or materials of medicine. All systems of medicine, based on drug therapies, have their own Materia medica. It is known by different names in different systems of medicine. It is termed as pharmacology in Allopathy, Dravya Guna in Ayurveda, Guna Padam in Siddha, and Materia Medica in Homeopathy. Pharmacology is based on physico-chemical properties of drug substances. Dravya Guna is based on Thridosa Sidhanda (vatha, pitha and kapha). Guna padam is based on Mucheer Amaippu (vatham, pitham, silatumam). Materia medica is based on dynamic properties of drugs applied on Law of Similars.

General Materia Medica

It is the body of collected knowledge about the therapeutic properties of any substance (drug) used for healing with their sources, preparations, doses, and use.

Homoeopathic Materia Medica

It is concerned with the study of homoeopathic drugs used in the treatment of patients. It is the record book of the effects of homeopathic drugs on human beings based on principles of drug proving on humans (Organon of Medicine 105-145). According to Hahnemann (Organon of Medicine 143,), "Homeopathic Materia Medica is a collection of real. pure, reliable mode of action of simple medicinal substances, a volume of book of nature". In other words it is an encyclopedia of purported therapeutic properties of each homeopathic preparation, which is ascribed through proving. Therefore, Materia medica acts as a prescribing reference guide and source for compiling Homeopathic repertory. In simple words Homeopathic Materia Medica is a book containing the systematic record of the drugs that are proved on healthy human beings of both sexes and different age groups.

It is the study of the action of drugs on healthy human being as a whole taking into consideration individual susceptibility and its reaction to various circumstances and time. In Homeopathic Material Medica, under each drug, a list of symptoms is mentioned according to parts of the body affected and generalities as unique modalities of the symptoms. A good prescription by a homoeopath mainly depends upon the case receiving, processing and a sound knowledge of Homoeopathic Materia Medica. Each drug in Materia Medica not only has its own personality with its mental and physical constitution but also has its own affinity to an area, direction, spread, tissue, organ, and system. Study of a drug in context of altered sensation, function and structure covers the pathology caused by it, which is also expressed in the pathogenesis of the drugs. Materia Medica also has symptoms from toxicological and clinical proving. All this knowledge is of utmost importance in order to apply the remedies in various clinical conditions. Homeopathic Materia Medica is constructed differently as it considers the study of the action of drugs on individual parts or systems of the body or on animal or their isolated organs, only a partial study of life process under such action.

Evolution of Homeopathic Materia medica

- *Cinchona officianalis* was the first drug proved in homeopathy by Dr Hahnemann himself.

Types of Materia Medica

Different authors have written various types of homeopathic Materia medicas and have presented drugs as per their views and ideas. Some of the books of Homeopathic Materia Medica are enumerated below (Patil, 1999).

- Materia Medica Pura – It was written by Dr. Hahnemann in two volumes. First volume was published in 1830 and second one in 1833. He proved 99 drugs in his life times and these books contains all the detail subjective and objective signs and symptoms of these drugs.
- Physiological Materia Medica – It is written by Dr.W.H.Burt. It contains physiological actions of the drugs given in systematic manner along with other drugs.
- Clinical Materia Medica – It is written by Dr.E.A.Farrington. It provides an understanding of the drugs in simple manner.
- Comparative Materia Medica – It is written by Dr. E.A.Farrington. The book provides details for differentiating two seemingly similar remedies.
- Condensed Materia Medica – It is written by Dr. Constantine Hering. The book contains maximum symptoms of maximum drugs.

- Key note type Materia Medica – It is written by Dr. Allen. It seems a referral type book and should be referred after grasping a thorough knowledge of the remedy.
- Lectures on Materia Medica – It is written by Dr. J. T.Kent. It is compilation of lecture notes of Dr. Kent on Materia Medica.
- A Manual of Pharmacodynamics – It is written by Dr. R. Huges. Pharmacodynamics of the drugs is given in this book.
- Homeopathic Materia Medica with repertory of Indian Drugs – It is written by Boericke. The book is written in anatomical schematic presentation along with a repertory.
- Encyclopedia of Pure Materia Medica – It is written by Dr. T.F.Allen . The book is in 12 volumes. Even a small trifle of a drug has been described in this book.
- Comparative Materia Medica – It is written by Dr. H. Gross. It is a valuable document on Materia medica of Homeopathy.
- Expressive Drug Picture of Homeopathy Materia Medica – It is written by Dr. R.K. Chauhan. The book is in two volumes. The drugs have been detailed and described in pictorial style.

Sources of Homeopathic Materia Medica

- Proving on healthy humans.
- Proving on healthy animals.
- Proving on plants.
- Clinical Observations.
- Accidental source.
- Toxicological Source.
- Chemical Source.
- Empirical source
- Doctrine of signature.

Example of Therapeutic Materia Medica

- Aconite (monkshood): fearful, sudden, seizures
- Apis (bee): swelling, allergic reaction, better cold applications, no thirst. Insect stings.
- Arsenicum album (white arsenic): toxic effects, especially on GIT; Parvo; always restless, chilly, thirsty.
- Belladonna (deadly nightshade): sudden, red, throbbing. Painful. Angry. Compulsive. Fevers. Seizures.

- Bryonia (wild hops): Movement makes pains worse, a grouchy bear. Arthritis.
- Cantharis (Spanish Fly): burns, burning pains, cystitis
- Carbo vegetabilis (charcoal): cold, blue, collapse, neonate resuscitation
- Causticum (lime/potassium mix): involuntary urination, weak muscles, warts, trembling, old age problems. Paralysis.
- Ferrum phos (phos of iron): early inflammation, fever, <right, night, cold, dry.
- Gelsemium (yellow jasmine): dull, droopy, drowsy, chilled. Diarrhea from anticipation. Cats pull hair from back.
- Hepar sulph (Calc. sulphide): pain, hyper sensitive, chilly, grouchy, smelly. Interdigital cysts, infected ears, abscesses
- Ignatia (St. Ignatius bean): grief and ailments from grief, paradoxical symptoms.
- Ipecacuanha (Ipecac root): nausea, vomiting, bleeding, with a clean tongue.
- Ledum (Marsh tea): punctures, insect bites, >cold applications, yet injury feels cold to touch. Lyme disease.
- Magnesia phosphorica: colic, cramps, >light pressure and bend double.
- Mercurius vivus (sol): drooling, offensive, mouth and rectum, < by cold and > by heat, thick and coated tongue.
- Natrum muriaticum (salt): ailments from grief, wants salt, thirsty, loners, worse at the seashore, suppressed grief. Bite owners when petted.
- Phosphorus: friendly, affectionate. Thirst for cold water. Bleeding. Vomiting.
- Pulsatilla nigricans (windflower): clinging. Bland discharges, >consolation, >open air, >cold. Thirstless. Female problems. Prostatitis.
- Rhus toxicodendron (Poison ivy): creaky gate, skin, restless, joints better from walking or motion.
- Rumex (Yellow Dock): coughs from going from warm to cold air, tickling, teasing cough < pressure, < cold, prevents sleep.
- Ruta graveolens (Rue-bitterwort): sprains, strains, bruised bones and eyes.
- Sarsaparilla: urinary tract problems. Has to stand up to urinate. Horses losing hair from manes.
- Silica (sand): abscesses. Foreign bodies. Chilly or can desire cold. Feline acne. Timid.

- Thuja (Arbor vitae tree): hair oily, grows slowly, ringworm. Fearful--hides, cringes, freaks out in cages, and does not want to be held, though is affectionate.

Materia Medica of Homeopathy

1. ***Human Homeopathy***

a) Pocket Manual of Homeopathic Materia Medica by William Boericke. 9th edition . Revised and Enlarged with the addition of repertory by Oscar E. Boericke, A.B. Reprint edition 2001. Indian Books and Periodicals Publishers, Karol Bagh, New Delhi.

b) Lotus Materia medica by Robin Murphy. 2nd Revised edition. B.Jain Publishers (P) Ltd., New Delhi.

2. ***Veterinary Homeopathy***

It is concerned with the study of homoeopathic drugs used in the treatment of animals. It is the record book of the effects of homeopathic drugs on animals based on principles of drug proving mainly on humans. The following books are available on Materia Medica of veterinary Homeopathy.

a) The Veterinary Pharmacopeia, Materia Medica, and Therapeutics-Primary Source Edition. By George Gresswell, 2013. Nabu Press

b) Therapeutics of Veterinary Homeopathy and Repertory. By B.P. Madrewar and Mathew Glencross, 1996 (ist Edn.), 1999 (2nd Edn.), 2010 5th Impression, B.Jain Publishers (P) Ltd, New Delhi

c) A Veterinary Materia Medicaand Clinical Repertory. By George Macleod, Revised edition 1992. C.W.Daniel, U.K.

d) Materia Medica, Nosodes, and Repertory of Veteruinary Homeopathy. By B.P.Madrewar and Mathew Glencross. Edition 2024. B. Jain Publishers (P) Ltd. New Delhi.

e) Veterinary Materia Medica and Theraputics. By Kenelm Winslow and A. Eichhorn. 1919. Digitized by the Internet Archrive in 2012. 8th edition revised. American Veterinary Publishing Company.

Description of Remedies in Boericke Materia Medica of Homeopathy

An example how remedies have been described in Pocket Manual of Homeopathic Materia Medica with Indian medicine and Repertory is given below.

Arnica (Leopard's Bane)

General : It produces symptoms similar to those resulting from injuries, septic conditions, apoplexy etc.

Mind: Fear touch, indifference, after mental strain or shock etc.

Head: Hot with cold body, confused, sensitivity of brain with sharp pinching pain etc.

Eyes: Retinal hemorrhage, bruished sore feeling, must keep eyes open etc.

Ears: Noises in ear, shooting in and around ears, blood from ears, dull hearing after concussion etc.

Nose: Bleeding after fits of coughing, sore nose etc.

Mouth: Fetid breath, dry thirsty , bitter taste, sore gums etc.

Face: Sunken, red, Herpes in face etc

Stomach: Distaste for milk and meat,, hunger, vomiting of blood pain during eating etc.

Abdomen: Distended, stiches under false rib etc.

Stool: Tenesmus in diarrhea, offensive brown bloodt stool, must lie down after every stool etc.

Urine:Retained from over-exertion, dark brick-red sediment, micturition etc.

Female: Bruised parts after labor, violent after-pains, mechanical uterine hemorrhage etc.

Respiratory: Cough depending on cardiac lesion,, acute tonsilitishoarseness, bloody expectoration etc.

Heart; Severe pain in elbow of left arm, feeling of stiches in heart, cardiac dropsy with distressing dyspnea etc.

Extremities: Gout, pain in back and limbs, fear of being touched etc.

Skin : Black, blue, itching, burning sensation, acne etc.

Sleep: Sleepless, restless, awaken with hot head, dream of death etc.

Fever: Febrile symptoms etc

Modalities: Worse, least touch; motion, rest etc.

Relationship: Antidote – Camph; Complementary – Acon, Ipec etc

Dose : Third to thirtieth potency etc.

Description of Remedies in Veterinary Homeopathy books

An example how remedies have been described in Veterinary Homeopathy is given below (Veterinary Homeopathy by P.K. Naveen, 2017, Pushpa Naveen Navaneeth, Chalakudy P.O. Thrissur District, Kerala, India.

Arnica Montana

Source: Arnica Montana, Leopard's-bane. Fallkraut etc.

General: Acts on muscular, serous, cellular tissues and tendons, producing conditions quite similar to those of injuries . Acts on capillaries, through motor nerves affects cerebrospinal axis, in digestive tract produces irritation etc.

Key Notes: Bruishing, trauma, pain, fear of being touched etc.

Clinical: Blunt force trauma, concussion, accident, injuries, post traumatic stress, nose bled etc.

Guiding Indications: Post operative rehabilitation, renowned traumatic injury, relieves hemorrhage in any part of the body including blood in milk, physical and mental shock, muscular tonic etc.

Relationship : Complemetary - Aco, Ipec, Verat.: Compatible- Acon. Apis, Nux, Phos etc.; Antidote- Calend, Cep, Ign etc.; Antidoted by- Aco, Ars, Camph Ign etc.

Modalities : Aggravation- Least touch, motion, rest, dampness; Amelioration – Lying down or with head low.

Remark- It appears to me that whatever is given in Veterinary Books has been extrapolated from Human Homeopathic Materia Medica as is clearly evident from the above example of *Arnic*a description.

Repertory

The Repertory is a book listing all of the symptoms for the homeopathic single remedies and is like an index for the Materia Medica which is full of information collected from toxicology, drug proving and clinical experiences. Each remedy has a set of symptoms associated with it and the Repertory assists in associating these two elements.

Need of the Repertory

Repertories serve as an instrument at the disposal of the physician for sifting through the maze of symptoms of the vast Homoeopathic Materia Medica. Repertories aim at simplifying the work of the physician to find the indicated remedy by eliminating the non-indicated remedies.

Repertorisation

The process of repertoriasation is essentially an elimination process, which starts with a broad choice and slowly narrows down the field, giving an adequate small group of medicine, so that the final selection is made easier with the help of further reference to the materia medica.

Classification of Repertories

There are number of repertories available in the market. Broadly repertories have been classified on the basis of i. over all appearance, ii. internal formatting and iii. group characteristics.

i. Over all appearance- This group has three types of repertories such as book repertories, card repertories and software packages.

ii. Internal formatting- There are two types of repertories (Puritan group and Logical Utilitarian group) on the basis of internal formatting.

   In Puritan group, purity of language of the drug proving is maintained. It is used for reference purpose. Repertories are analogues to the index of the symptoms as they are presented in the Materia Medica. Example- Kneer repertory, Gentry's repertory.

   Logical Utilitarian group has distinct principles. The symptoms may not be found in the language of the materia medica. The form of the symptoms is changed to fit in to the arrangement of the repertories. Example Kent's repertory.

iii. Group characteristics classification is most pragmatic. General repertories, regional repertories, particular repertories, alphabetical repertories, concordance repertories ,comparative repertories ,pathogenic repertory ,reference repertories, card repertories, computer repertories and therapeutic digest are in this group.

General Repertories

The general repertories are logical utilitarian repertories and are useful for individualization. They facilitate the adaption of general symptom for repertorisation. They have three groups based on i. deductive logic ,ii. inductive logic and iii. Clinical.

Generals symptoms are given prime importance in deductive repertories. The analysis of the case for these repertories is also based on the premise of the deductive logic, where the generals symptoms are given higher ranking than the particular symptoms. Example. Kent's repertory, Synthesis. Principles of deductive logic are adopted by synthetic repertory but do not include particular symptoms.

Repertories based on inductive logic means from particulars to general symptoms. In these repertories the different elements of a symptom like location, sensation modality and concomitants can be brought together on the basis of certain constants and a general symptom can be constructed. That is called a Synthetic general. A particular sensation expressed at more than two location at any given time, it can be elevated to the level of a general symptom, provided the modalities remain the same for all the locations expressing that sensation. If a concomitant is also present the generalization become stronger.

Clinical repertories have many clinical rubrics under different systems, and the medicines are given against the name of the disease. Similar to general repertories, the clinical repertories also cover the therapeutic information for the whole of the organism and come under logical utilitarian group. The construction of these repertories affords the flexibility of adopting either the deductive or inductive logic at any given time, and highly useful when there is a significant amount of clinical data available in a case. Example . Clinical repertory by J.H. Clark

Homeopathic Pharmacy

The word 'pharmacy' implies the place where the medicines are prepared and distributed. Homeopathic pharmacy is the art and science of collecting, compounding, combining, preparing, preserving and standardizing drugs and medicines according to the homoeopathic principles; and also dispensing medicines or remedies according to the prescriptions of homeopaths. Homeopathic pharmacy is different from conventional pharmacy. Homeopathic pharmacy differs from conventional pharmacy in sources of drug, collection of drug, preparation, dosage forms.

Homoeopathic pharmacy is based on theory of dynamization and drugs get entry in homoeopathy after complete proving. Homeopathic pharmacy provides information about sources of drugs, collection of drug, drug preparation, drug action, drug proving, method of quality testing, standardization, storage, dispensing, and administration as well as legislation in relation to homoeopathic pharmacy and pharmaceutical industry. Homeopathic pharmacy emphasizes the concept of drug proving and drug dynamization, and on evolution and relationship of homoeopathic pharmacy to Organon of Medicine and Materia Medica. It also includes the elementary history of botany, zoology and chemistry with rules of their nomenclature and their respective terminologies. Further it also includes the study of modes of administration of medicines and posology.

Pharmacopeia and Homeopathic Pharmacopeia

Pharmacopeia

The term pharmacopeia has been derived from ancient Greek: φαρμακοποιία, romanized: pharmakopoiia "making of (healing) medicine, drug-making» -ία -ia. A pharmacopeia, (meaning "drug-making"), in its modern technical sense, is a book containing directions for the identification of compound medicines, and published by the authority of a government or a medical or pharmaceutical society (Morrel, 1911). Pharmacopeia is made up of two words i.e. pharmakon and poieen meaning 'drug' and 'to make' respectively. Pharmacopeias provide standards for pharmaceutical substances and medicinal products. Standards are an important tool in the regulation of the quality of medicines.

Homeopathic Pharmacopeia

Homeopathic pharmacopeia is a supreme authoritative book, published by an authority, govt. of any country that contains a list of drugs used in homeopathy, approved by an authority, and deals with the rules and regulations of standardization of drug substances. Homeopathic pharmacopeia are of two types such as official (published by an authority such as government of the country, medical or pharmaceutical society) or unofficial (published by any person other the authority).

Homeopathic Pharmacopeia contains list of drugs with information on source, habitat, description, identification, collection, preparation, preservation, combining, compounding, standardization and posology etc.

Evolution of Homeopathic Pharmacopeia

- In 1805, S. Hahnemann announced his new method of pharmacological process in a treatise: Fragmenta de Viribus Medicamentorum Positives Sive in Sino Corpore.
- In 1825, Carl W. Casperi published first Homeopathic Pharmacopeia in Germany.
- Dr. Hartmann, translated the first Homeopathic pharmacopeia in Latin and it was reprinted in England in 1829.
- A new Homeopathic Pharmacopeia with posology and administration of homeopathic doses was brought out by Jahr in 1942.
- In 1845, Gruner of Dresden introduced some technical improvements and recommended precipitating metal for their trituration.
- In 1845, Schmidt recommended water instead of alcohol for preparing 1st attenuation from acids in his pharmacopeia. He also advised to prepare attenuation of phosphorus from tincture.

- In 1852, Dr. Buchner published a pharmacopeia describing the mode of preparing homeopathic medicine.
- In 1870, British Homeopathic society published British Homeopathic Pharmacopeia accepted as standard for homeopathy.
- In 1892, first Indian Homeopathic Pharmacopeia was published by M. Bhattacharya and company. Its 14th edition has come in 1980.
- In 1897 American Homeopathic Pharmacopeia was published by American Homeopathic Society.
- In 1898, Homeopathic Pharmacopeia of France was published. It ran into several editions. New drugs in the categories of nosodes, organs, tissues, biochemicals/organochemicals and minerals were included.
- In 1901, Homeopathic Pharmacopeia of United States appeared with the concept of uniform drug strength of 10%.
- In 1971, First volume of Homeopathic Pharmacopeia of India was published by the Ministry of Health and Family welfare, Government of India. So far 10 volumes of Homeopathic pharmacopeia of India has been published in different years.
- Veterinary Homeopathic Pharmacopeia of India is in the process of compilation and publication.

Homeopathic Pharmacopeia of India

- First volume of Homeopathic Pharmacopeia of India was published in 1971 by the Ministry of Health and Family welfare, Government of India. In which standards for the preparation of homeopathic drugs in the country have been laid down. So far 10 volumes of Homeopathic pharmacopeia of India has been published in different years (1971, 1974, 1978, 1984, 1987, 1990, 1999, 2000, 2006 and 2013). There are total 1111 monographs has been published in ten volumes by the Council. A combined document of volume I to V and another of VI to IX have been published in 2016 by Government of India, Ministry of Health and Family Welfare Department of Ayurveda, Yoga and Naturopathy, Unani, Siddha and Homeopathy, New Delhi.
- It is the official book of standards of homeopathic medicines in terms of schedule II of the Drugs and Cosmetics Act 1940 and Rules, 1945.
- The Indian manufacturers are legally bound to manufacture Homeopathic medicines as per standards and methodology given in the Homeopathic Pharmacopeia of India.

- If the standards of some drugs are not given in Homeopathic Pharmacopeia of India, manufacturers are free to undertake manufacturing as per any recognized Pharmacopeia of the other country.
- Homeopathic Pharmacopeia of India is prepared by the Homeopathic Pharmacopeia Committee constituted by the Government of India.

Present State of Homeopathic Pharmacopeia in the world

- Homeopathic Pharmacopeia of India (HPI), 10 volumes (1971 to 2013).
- Homeopathic Pharmacopeia of United States, year 1897 revised in 2016.
- National homeopathic pharmacopoeias have been developed and published also in countries such as Germany, United Kingdom, France, Brazil and Mexico.

References

Morel, H.E.l (1911). "Pharmacopoeia". In Chisholm, Hugh (ed.). Encyclopædia Britannica. Vol. 21 (11th ed.). Cambridge University Press. pp. 353–355.

Munir Ahmed : Introduction to Repertorisation

Mohanty : Text book of Repertories

Patil, J.D. (1999). Gems of Homeopathic Materia Medica. B.Jain Publisher (P) Ltd., New Delhi.

www.ccrhindia.org/drugproving.asp

www.homeopathyeurope.org/publications/guidelines/homeopathic-provings

https://asia.nikkei.com/Business/Technology/Homeopathy-India-s-traditional-system-of-medicine

Tiwari : Essentials of repertorisation

11

Understanding Constitution, Psychology and Behavior

Constitution

The word 'constitution' is derived from a Latin word "Constituere" that means to set up or to make up or to establish. Therefore, it is the structure, composition, physical make up or nature of something consisting inherited qualities modified by environment. Constitution in homeopathy is defined as the physical and mental makeup which is expressed through physical built, characteristics, desires, aversions, reaction including emotional and intellectual attributes. In other words constitution incorporates the individual's combined physical body type (including nervous system and metabolism), mental thinking, style, emotional reactivity and temperament.

Classification of constitution

Human constitution has been classified in different ways in different systems of health care.

Chinese concept- Constitution has been classified as Yang and Yin.

Ayurveda concept- Constitution has been classified as Vatha, Pitha, Kapha.

*Hippocratic conc*ept- Constitution has been classified as short and thick; and long and thin.

Physical appearance concept -On the basis of physical appearance, constitution has been classed as short and thick; and long and thin.

Humour concept- Constitution has been classified as sanguine, choleric, phlegmatic and melancholic.

Bazin concept- Constitution has been classified as scrofulous, gouty and syphilitic.

Vanniers and Zissus concept-Constitution has been classified as phosphoric (tall, thin, delicate, easy tiring, yellow teeth dislike hard work, orderly and fastidious person), Fluoric (unbalanced, irregular body, obtuse angle of outstretched arms, irregular teeth, untidy, cunning, unreliable) and Carbonic (mentally and physically up right person having square white teeth, orderly, responsible and capable person).

*Dr. Eduard von Grauvogl con*cept- He (a German Homeopath) has classified constitution as carbo-nitrogenoid, oxygenoid and hydrogenoid constitution based on different biochemical contents of the body.

i. Carbo-nitrogenoid constitution- There is an excess of carbon and nitrogen. Physical characteristics are marked by obesity followed by emaciation in later stage, dirty and unhealthy skin with offensive perspiration, dry brittle nails with longitudinal striation.

ii. Oxygenoid constitution- There is an excess of oxygen. Physical characteristics are marked by lean, thin, cachectic body prone to self-destruction and ulceration, rickety, anemic, enlarged lymph node, elegant round fingers, beautiful long nail with white spots.

iii. Hydrogenoid constitution- There is an xcess of hydrogen. Physical characteristics are marked by obese, round, short limbed, swollen bodily appearance; edematous, cold and humid hands; and clammy skin.

Ernst Kretschner concept – Constitution has been classified as Asthenic (frail, linear physique, lean narrow built, poor skin secretion, narrow shoulder, narrow flat chest, sharp rib angle, and thin stomach), Athletic (strong bone, muscles and skin, middle size with projecting shoulders, superb chest), Dysplastic (irregular) and Pyknik (plump physique).

Psychology

'Psychology' is defined as the science of behavior (humans or animals) in relation to environment. Human behavior is nothing but only an expression or response. It includes the study of conscious, sub-conscious and unconscious behaviour. Psychology is concerned with 'how' and 'why' of conduct and of thinking. The basic purpose of psychology is to understand the behavior in scientific manner. Human behavior is extraordinarily complex and is influenced by different factors. In homeopathy, a knowledge of psychology is essential to understand and analyze the patient in a better way by incorporating the mental and physical aspects of the patient.

Hahnemann integrated his understanding of theology, philosophy and psychology into" The Organon of the Healing Art." The main sections on homoeopathic psychology and the treatment of mental disorders are described in aphorisms 210 to 230. Mourning and grief are extinguished in the emotional mind on hearing an account of another's still greater bereavement, even if the account is only fictitious.

Mind is the parent of all desires. An illness may be primarily physical or psychological, it is always the disorder of the whole person-not just the lungs or psyche. Fatigue or cold lowers tolerance for psychological stress, leading to emotional upset and in turn lowering resistance to physical disease. In short, the individual is psychobiological with the environment. Hahnemann introduced the subject of homoeopathic psychology in the Materia Medica Pura and The Spirit of the Homeopathic Medical Doctrine (1813). Most interesting is Hahnemann's application of the homoeopathic principles of similars to cure by psychology (Vide Materia Medica Pura, page 15).

Modern psychology views the mind of an individual in three categories as emotions, will and understanding. The homeopathic principles hold the key to a deeper study of psychology than is commonly understood. Sympathy and similars can go a long way in the realms of the psyche. The combination of homeopathic psychology and mesmerism represents a largely unexplored region of the Organon of the Healing Art.

Behavior

Behavior is the range of action and mannerism made by the individuals in conjunction with themselves or their environment. It is observable activities of humans and animals. It is anything observable a human or animal does. The term behavior includes all motor activities, cognitive activities and affective activities. In another words human behavior is an expressed and potential capacity for physical, mental and social activities, that are influenced by variety of factors (attitude, authority, culture , environment, ethics, genetics, moral and perception etc) , during the phases of life. Common human behaviors include conflict, communication, cooperation, creativity, social interaction, tradition and work.

Expression of Behavior

- Behavior is expressed through actions, gestures and movements .

Types of Human Behavior

- Assertive- It is a positive self-affirmation valuing other persons also.
- Avoidance- It is a conscious/unconscious defense trying to escape from unpleasant situations or feeling (anxiety and pain).
- Submissive- It is submission to someone else's will putting his own desires lower than others. This type of behavior help in reducing anxiety, guilt or fear.
- Aggressive behavior- It is communicated verbally or non-verbally. Such people may invade the personal space of the others.

Factors Influencing the Human Behavior

- Biological factors (hormones from adrenals, pancreas, thyroid).
- Social factors (interpersonal such as person's social support network relations with other peoples, person's religious or spiritual relations; institutional factors such as rules, regulations and informal structures existing in organization or community or society; community factors such as environment and resources available in the community; and public policy).

Animal Behavior

- As per Britannica, the concept of animal behavior refers to everything that animal do (movement, and other activities) in response to a stimulus. Blinking, eating, walking, vocalizing, huddling, defecating, urinating, standing etc. are the example of animal behavior.
- It is the result of biology and environment.
- It is the change in the activity of an animal in response to an stimulus
- Behavioral changes are triggered by an internal or external stimulus or cue.
- The animal behavior fall in to two categories such as innate and learned. The former ones are uncontrolled and automatic. While later ones are to be taught. Instinct , imprinting, conditioning and imitation have bearing on behavior.
- Goats are more reactive and aggressive.
- Sheep are more fearful and shy.

Types of Animal Behavior

Animals show following type of behavior.

- Feeding Behavior
- Social behavior
- Sexual behavior
- Parental behavior
- Drinking behavior
- Excretory behavior
- Exploratory behavior
- Conflict behavior
- Sleep behavior
- Aggressive behavior

- Submissive behavior
- Fear behavior
- Cattle show play, nutritional, social, reproductive, locomotive and resting behaviors.

Behavioral Needs of Farm Animals

The major behavioral needs of farm animals are enumerated below

- Reaction to danger (flight and escape)
- Ingestion
- Body care (including elimination)
- Motion
- Exploration/territorialism
- Rest
- Association (including social and reproductive behavior)

***Needs Related to Avoidance of Adverse conditions* (Webster, 1987)**

- Freedom from thirst
- Freedom from hunger
- Freedom from malnutrition
- Freedom from prolonged discomfort
- Freedom from injury, disease, fear and stress

Abnormal Behavior of Farm Animals

- Stereotyped Behaviors- Stereotyped behaviors such as bar- biting, tongue rolling, swinging the tongue from side to side outside mouth, or rolling the tongue inside the mouth seen on feeding of inadequate roughage in artificially suckled calves are seen in farm animals . Tongue playing is believed to be the result of long term frustration caused by suppressed suckling and feeding, and a boring environment (Seo *et al.*, 1998a,b).
- Injurious Behaviors- Behaviors that cause injuries to other animals are common when animals are housed in deficient environment. Injurious behaviors are not so common in cattle as in pigs and poultry. Excessive self grooming is another injurious behavior.
- Redirected Behaviors- Where the motivation for a behavioral need is particularly strong and is thwarted by environmental insufficiency, animals may attempt to redirect the motivation to the performance of a

similar behavior. This is especially common with ingestion. An abnormal diet will often precipitate abnormal oral behaviours, and deficiencies of fibre, phosphorus and sodium will produce cravings for the nutrient,or pica.

Differences between Human and Animal Mental Symptoms

- Animals do not have reflective consciousness. It is specially developed function of human mind. Animals show their mental symptoms directly from the unconscious mind. Animals' mental symptoms can be equated to what is in the mental section of the repertory that is a direct expression in the same way – the emotions, the cravings, the aversions. Specific human events such as "explanations" or "repression" (unconscious blocking of unpleasant emotions, impulses, memories and thought from conscious mind) are not available for use in animals .
- Animals have a simple memory (a function of the unconscious mind) somewhat different than ours. We can make the conscious effort to recollect a memory while memory returns automatically (eidetic memory- not recalled in usual sense) in animals when encountering a stimulus (present at the time of the event).
- Animals don't have repression and they are not caught in a sense of time or by making symbols of what happens. Everything is immediate, a continuous "now".
- In human homeopathic practice , patients reveal themselves (speak without guiding) giving more "direct" information . It avoids the tendency to speculate and give false reasons for the behavior. The animals should be observed in their more natural expressions to get information directly rather than when they are restrained or controlled by circumstances.
- The animals show direct and immediate symptoms based on present stimuli as they do not have a sense of time (do not project into the future or dwell on the past).
- Care must be exercised in applying human-derived symptoms to animals as animals do not project pattern of mental symptoms of conscious mind.
- Animal experience differs from the human even in same environment. Therefore, it is erroneous to consider animals just like humans.
- Emotion shown by an animal may sometimes be a husbandry issue rather than a homeopathic case. For example, aggression shown by a dog in a yard on approaching by a stranger is their normal response rather than an emotion. Observations should be taken, without interpretation, directly

to the most reliable rubric. Translation of behavior into rubric is very important aspect.

- It is advisable to work with physical symptoms first. Then bring the mental symptoms to refine.

References

Seo, T., Sato, S., Kosaka, K., Sakamoto, N., Tokumoto, K. and Katoh, K. (1998a). Development of tongue-playing in artificially reared calves: effects of offering a dummy-teat, feeding of short cut hay and housing system. Applied Animal Behaviour Science, 56, 1–12.

Seo, T., Sato, S., Kosako, H., Sukamoto, K., Tokumoto, K. and Kakah, K. (1998b).Tongue-playing and heart rate in calves. Applied Anim. Behaviour Sci. 58:179–182.

Webster, A.J.F. (1987). Understanding the Dairy Cow, pp. 330–332. BSP Professional Books, Oxford.

12

Principles of Management of Animal Diseases with Special Reference to Homeopathy

Homoeopathy is a different system of health care with a holistic, logical and philosophical tailor made approach in the treatment of an individual. The principles of management of diseases or treatment of diseases using homeopathy in animals are in no way different from that of human homeopathy. Homeopathy has potential to cure both human and animal diseases.

Homeopathic Philosophy or Principles

Management of diseases of humans or animals using homeopathy is based on eight basic principles or philosophies.

1. ***Similia Similibus Curentur***- The basic philosophy of homeopathy is based on the 'Similia Similibus Curentur' (Latin) or Law of similars (like cures like) , natural law of healing. Which states that a disease can be cured by a drug or substance which is capable of producing similar symptoms in healthy subject when given in minute doses. The treatment in homeopathy is based on the similarity of symptoms of the patient to those of a drug described in Homoeopathic Materia Medica. Drug selection is based not only on the similarity of the presenting symptom, but also on modalities, constitution and temperament of the patient and exciting and fundamental causes.
2. ***Principle of Individualization***- Individualization is the process of differentiating one individual from others of the same group by some peculiar or unique features. No two individuals in this world are alike. Therefore, the disease affecting them will not be alike or similar. The medicines used to cure the same disease in different subjects are different. Therefore the treatment should be based on individual's characteristics. Be it an animal or human.
3. ***Law of Simplex***- It stresses on the use of only one single homeopathic drug at a time. Basically there is no place for poly pharmacy in

homeopathy. Dr. Hahnemann writes in aphorism 247 “it is wrong to attempt to employ complex means when single means suffice”. In aphorism 272 he states that only one single simple medicinal substance should be administered in a given case at a time. Homeopathic remedies are proved singly. If more than one remedy is given, the pure effect of the remedy can not be appreciated. Vital force governing the body is single and dynamic.

4. ***Law of Minimum***- Homeopathic drugs should be used in minimal or small doses to stimulate the human or animal to produce perceptible change. It finds support from ‘Arndt-Schulz ‘ rule ,according to that weak stimuli accelerate vital process, moderate stimuli promote vital process, and strong stimuli suppress vital process. Drugs given in minimum dose have advantage of avoiding unwanted aggravation.
5. ***Principle of Drug-proving***- Homoeopathy stresses upon human experimentation. Drug proving is done on healthy subjects. The homeopathic drug is given in minute dose to a good number of healthy humans of both sexes and the symptoms produced by the drug in healthy subject are observed and recorded. Such proving can also be done on animals. But most of the proving have been done on healthy humans. The fine symptoms that a homoeopathic physician looks for in a patient: mental and emotional symptoms, precise subjective sensations, modalities etc., cannot be available or appreciated in animal experimentation. Therefore, drug proving is mostly and usually done in healthy humans.
6. ***Principle of Drug-dynamization***- In homeopathy, potentized drugs are used and the drug is not prescribed on physiological dose as in allopathy. Homeopathic potentization is done through sequential dilution and succussion. The process of potentization increases the power and the effect of the drug. It is mathematico-mechanical process by virtue of which the inherited dormant dynamic curative power of the drugs is aroused or increased through simultaneous and successive process of dilution and succussion in definite order.
7. ***Principle of Chronic diseases***- Hahnemann wrote in Aphorism 78 of 6th edition of Organon, “The true natural chronic diseases are those that arise from a chronic miasm (From Greek Miasma meaning Fault or Taint, and may be inherited or acquired), which when left to themselves, and unchecked by the employment of those remedies that are specific for them, always go on increasing and growing worse, notwithstanding the best mental and corporeal regimen, and torment the patient to the

end of his life with ever aggravated sufferings. "All those diseases occurring due to faulty lifestyles, unhealthy environment or various medications (Iatrogenic diseases) are not a part of this group of diseases. Homoeopathy considers chronic diseases to be a faulty functioning of the vital force under the influence of chronic miasm, due to which series of illnesses/ symptom complexes develop and can be cured only with a constitutional (anti-miasmatic) remedy.

8. ***Principle of Vital Force***- Vital force a triune entity consisting body, mind and spirit. It is super sensual thing which animates the material body in a harmonic way maintaining the normal physiology of the living body. Dr. Hahnemann described the concept of vital force (in the 9th–17th aphorisms) in the Organon of Medicine. He said that material organism, without vital force , is capable of no sensation ,no function, no self-preservation; it derives all sensation and performs all the functions of life solely by means of immaterial being(the vital principle) which animates the material organism in health and in disease. In the sixth edition of the Organon of Medicine, he replaced the word vital force with vital principle (10th aphorism of the sixth edition). Vital force and vital principle have different meanings; force means energy, whereas principle means a fundamental truth or proposition that serves as the foundation for a system of belief or behavior or a chain of reasoning. Homoeopathy believes in the existence of a force, which animates the human organism and the harmonious functioning of the body is because of its equilibrium.

References

Hahnemann, S. (2004). Organon of Medicine (5th and 6th combined ed). New Delhi: B Jain Publishers; 2004 (Google Scholar).

Noble, D. (2016). Dance to the Tune of Life: Biological Relativity (1st ed). Cambridge, UK: Cambridge University Press; 2016. (Google Scholar).

13

Mastitis and Mammary Diseases

Mastitis

Mastitis is an economically important disease of dairy animals (cows and buffaloes) caused by a wide variety of pathogens (bacteria, some viruses, fungi).Major pathogens are *Streptococcus agalactiae*, *Staphylococcus aureus, E. coli, Streptococcus uberis, Str. Dysagalactiae, Campylobactor*, *Corynebacterium pyogenes*, *Klebsiell*a spp. *Pasteurella*, *Pseudomona*s, *Mycoplasma*, *Enterobactor*, *Trichosporon* spp., *Aspergillus fumigatus*, *Candida* spp., *Leptospira* spp. and many more. Mastitis is also seen in lactating goats and sheep. As compared to ruminants mastitis is less common in bitches. Mastitis is an inflammatory disease of the udder parenchyma irrespective of its etiology. The disease occurs in clinical and subclinical forms. Clinical mastitis is of two types viz. acute mastitis and chronic mastitis. Subclinical mastitis is characterized by an increased number of somatic cells (>100,000 cells/ml) and/or pathogens in the milk with no apparent clinical change in the udder and milk. While clinical mastitis is associated with local (hot, pain full swelling of the udder) and general symptoms along with change in milk (increased cell count, increased pathogens, physical and chemical changes in the milk). Antibiotics (local and systemic) are principally used to combat infection in modern medicine. Their erratic use has led to the emergence of bacterial resistance (Wallmann 2016; Schulz-Stübner 2016). In organic and biodynamic farming, the use of antibiotics is restricted by legal requirements supporting the use of alternative and complementary therapies. Homeopathy is most popular alternative, complimentary holistic approach in health care throughout world (European Union 2008). It is being used by ecological and biodynamic farmers in animal husbandry (León *et al.* 2006; Gordon *et al.*, 2012). This unique mode of treatment, a brain child of Dr. Hahnemann, is based on principle of similia, drug proving (human volunteers),and potentization (dilution and succession). Homeopathic remedies are potentiated drugs of plants or minerals origin tested on healthy human provers and the same drugs are being used on animals as rarely any homeopathic drug has been tested on animals (Ekert, 2013).

Clinical Characteristics of Mastitis

- Clinical mastitis (Fig. 1) may occur in per acute, acute or chronic forms.
- Change in size, shape, consistency , color, and temperature of mammary glands depends on the severity of the mastitis and its causative agent.
- Change in mammary secretion (physical, chemical, cellular and microbial changes in milk)
- Systemic reaction (fever, toxemia, tachycardia, rumen atony, depression, recumbency, anorexia).
- Acute mastitis (Fig. 1) is clinically characterized by hot, swollen , painful udder with or without systemic reaction.
- Chronic mastitis (Fig. 1) is clinically characterized by hard indurated udder.

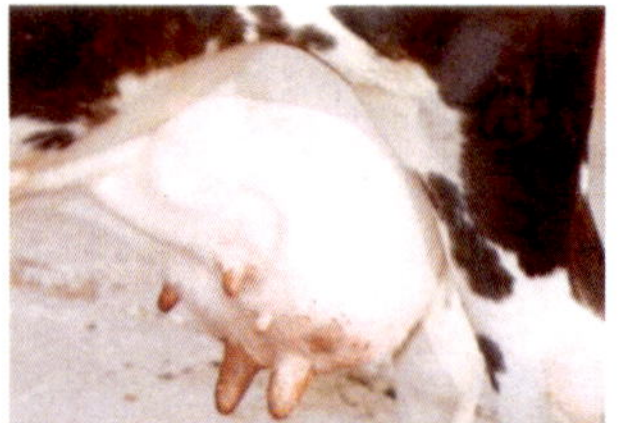
Acute mastitis

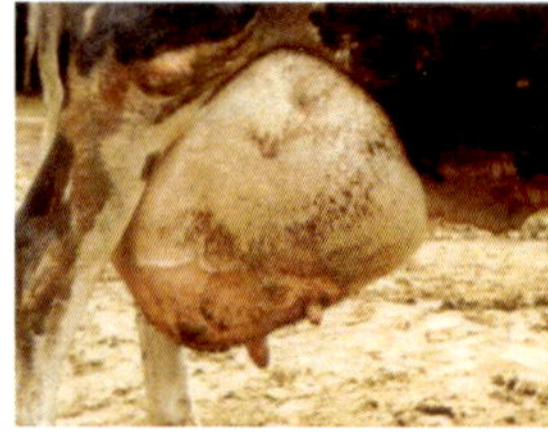
Fibrosed mastitis

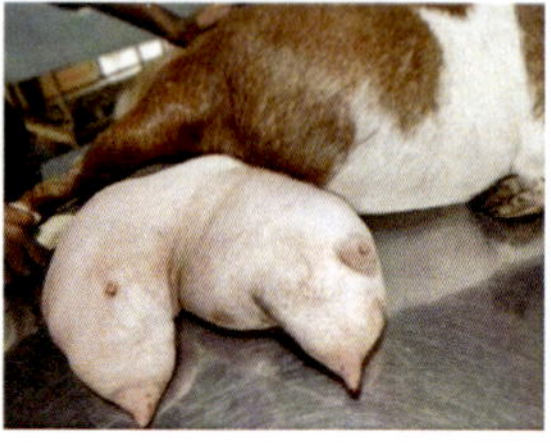
Acute mastitis in goat

Fig. 1. Mastitis in cows and goat. Note physical changes in udder.

Clinical Characteristics of Sub-clinical Mastitis

- High somatic count in the milk
- No visible changes in milk
- No apparent changes in the udder.

Treatment of Mastitis

- In modern medicine, antibiotics are the drug of choice for treatment and prevention.
- Over reliance and erratic use of antibiotics has led to the emergence of resistance, a major cause of treatment failure as well as residual problem of antibiotics in the milk searching for an effective, ecofriendly alternative medicines.
- Homeopathy is widely accepted as an alternative or complimentary therapeutic approach.

Homeopathic Drugs in the Management of Mastitis

- Homeopathic medicines seem to provide an effective alternative treatment option.The drugs can be used in 30 C potency three to four times a day till clinical, bacteriological and cellular recovery. Single drug therapy or homeopathic combination remedies can be used.
- Frequent stripping is a valuable treatment adjunct.
- *Belladonna*- It is indicated in acute mastitis with red, hard/ tender swollen udder. Symptoms aggravated by touch, motion or pressure. The drug can also be given in cases of post-partum mastitis.
- *Apis mellifica*- It is indicated in cases of edematous, red and hot udder with hard swelling (shiny and of rosy color) & decreased thirst. Symptoms aggravated by heat and pressure and relieved by cold application.
- *Conium maculatum*- It is indicated in mastitis with engorged mammary gland and stony induration, or udder with contusion / trauma or chronic mastitis.
- *Bryonia alba*- It is indicated in animals with swollen, hard, hot, painful, indurated mammary glands. In acute condition, pain is aggravated by motion but relieved by pressure and lying down. Bryonia animals are commonly observed lying on the inflamed portion of the udder.
- *Arnica montana*- It is indicated when mastitis is the result of injury to udder and blood in milk is seen. Symptoms aggravation by touch and motion and relieved by lying down.
- *Phytolacca*- It is a most common homeopathic remedy that is indicated in chronic as well as acute cases of mastitis with heavy, hard, stony, swollen, bluish red udder; watery, fetid mammary secretion; curdled milk with clot in acute phase; or small clots in chronic phase of the disease. The animal may resent washing and stripping.
- *Silicea*- It is the drug of choice in chronic mastitis caused by *Corynebacterium pyogenes* with multiple abscessation and bloody mammary discharge. Symptoms aggravation by cold and dampness.
- *Urtica urens*- It is indicated in acute mastitis with edema extending to perineal area, serous mammary discharge, decreased mammary secretion after parturition.
- Topical massage with *Arnica, Phytolacca* ointment in acute cases and with *Bryonia* ointment in in chronic cases.
- In a blind randomized control trial Keller and Sundrum (2018) observed that the effectiveness of individualised homeopathy does not go beyond

a placebo effect and successful treatment is highly dependent on the specific mastitis pathogen.

Use of Homeopathic Combination Remedies in the Management of Mastitis

- Dolisovet (a homeopathic combination remedy *containing Belladonna 1dH, Calendula MT, Echinacea* 1dH, *Dulcamar*a 1cH in ointment form for intramammary use) has shown beneficial therapeutic effect in the early stages of mastitis in restoring udder health and function. (Aubry *et al.*, 2013).
- Healwell VT6 – Sintex Internation Ltd (homeopathic combination remedy consisting of *Phytolcca* 200c, *Calcarea fluorica* 200c, *Silicea* 30c, *Belladonna* 30c, *Bryonia* 30c, *Arnica* 30c, *coniu*m 30c and *Ipecacuanh*a 30c in equal proportion given at the dose rate 10 pills four times daily until clinical resolution) has shown promising results in the management of udder diseases of riverine buffaloes (Varshney and Ram Naresh, 2004), and cows (Varshney and Ram Naresh, 2005).

Use of Homeopathy in Mastitis Prevention

- For mastitis prevention a combined nosode (containing five pathogen) was tested by Day (1986). He observed that as compared to 25 % placebo controlled animals, only 2.5 % animals treated with nosode developed mastitis.
- In another study, homeopathy was compared with internal teat sealer at drying off (Klocke *et al.*, 2010). Though there was mastitis protection in cows treated with homeopathy but the difference between both groups were non-significant.
- A trial of nosode (a combination of nosodes with *Streptococcinum, Staphylococcinum, Pyrogenium*, and *Escherichia coli* at a potency of 200c once daily for 5 days) in dairy cows with acute mastitis offered no additional effect as compared to placebo (Ebert *et al.*, 2017).
- A trial with a homeopathic combination remedy over five days in one group and single homeopathic treatment with homeopathic nosode (Tuberculinum) in other group of sub clinical mastitis along with placebo and untreated control showed no significant difference as far as bacteriological cure and somatic cell count was concerned (Klocke *et al.* 2007).

Thelitis

It is an inflammation of the teat usually associated with teat injury (Fig.2). It is different from mastitis and intractable to intramammary antibiotics.

Clinical Characteristics of Thelitis

- Sudden swelling on teats (Fig. 2)
- Teats are swollen, hot and painful
- Cistern wall not thickened
- Milking painful
- No change in physical and chemical properties of milk
- Negative White side test

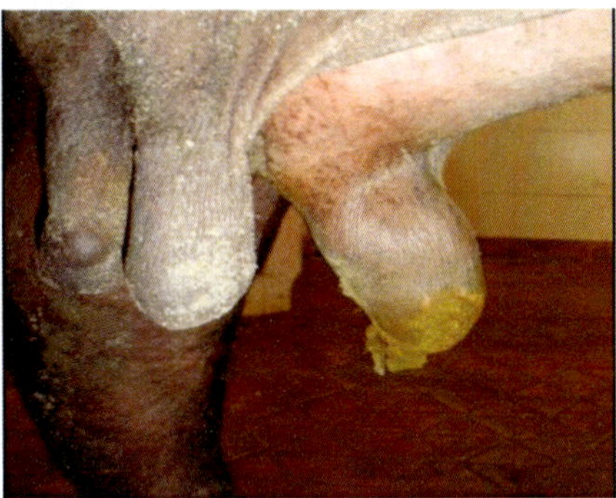

Fig. 2. Cow with Theilitis . Note there is teat injury.

Homeopathic Treatment

The following treatment has shown great promise in the treatment of thelitis (Varshney, 2006).

- Arnica 30c 10 pills PO TID on day 1st
- Bryonia 30c 10pills PO TID for next 2-3 days
- Bryonia cream (8% v/w) external application from day 1 for 2-3 days

Vesicular and Pustular Eruptions on Teats of FMD Affected Cows

Vesicular and pustular eruptions on the teats and its orifice of cows affected with FMD expose the animals to mastitis and make the milking painful and difficult. Secondary bacterial invasions may interfere with healing and lead to involvement of deeper tissues.

Clinical Characteristics

- Inappetance
- Watery nasal discharge
- Increased salivation and saliva hanging in long ropy strings
- Body temperature variable (102.0-104.0 ^{0}F)

- Lameness
- Foot lesions
- Varying size vesicles (1.5-2.0 cm) and/or pustular eruptions on the surface of the teats (Fig.3)
- Negative White side test

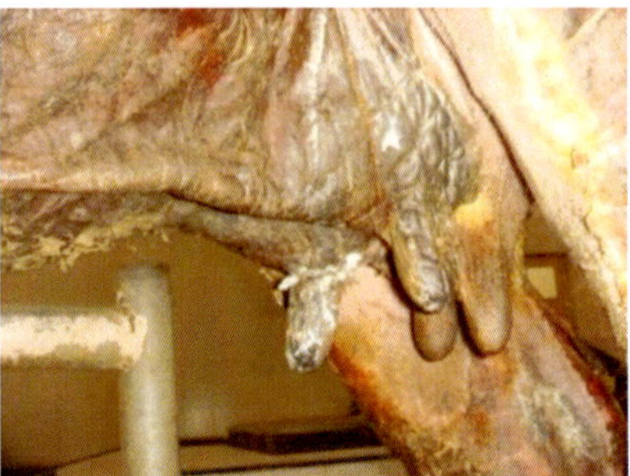

Fig. 3. FMD affected cow showing vesicular and pustular lesions on the teat.

Homeopathic Treatment

The following treatment has shown great promise in the treatment of vesicular and pustular FMD lesions (Varshney, 2007).

- Mercurius solubilis 30c 15 pills PO TID for 4 days
- Topical application of Calendula cream (4 g %) BID to TID
- Mercurius and Calendula have been described as antisyphilic remedy and excellent healing agent for open wounds respectively (Boericke, 2001). Signs of Mercurious solubilis are characterized by aphthae, salivation, vesicular and pustular eruptions with a tendency to suppurate in humans (Murphy, 2002).

Udder Edema

It is common in high producing dairy cows immediately before or after parturition. The disorder has many predisposing factors right from antepartum diet (excessive salt), age at first calving (older heifer are at risk), obesity, lack of exercise to nutrition. Udder edema is a risk factor for mastitis. Its etiology is uncertain. It may be associated with reduced mammary blood flow and increased intravenous pressure. It may be physiological or chronic

Clinical Characteristics

- Edema (soft, painless, swelling with pitting) is localized ventrally (Fig.4)
- It may extend to subcutaneous space around the udder and navel

- Acute physiological edema not painful
- Edema symmetrical in udder before parturition
- Midline fluid accumulation may be extending to the brisket
- It is common in heifers
- Edema is pitting on pressure
- It usually resolve within a week of parturition.
- In many cases it remain persisting through out lactation.
- There is no alteration in milk
- White side mastitis test remains negative

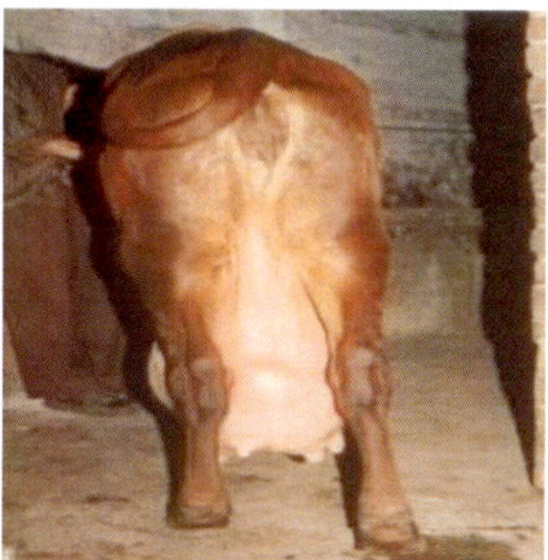

Fig. 4. Cow with udder edema showing edematous udder.

Homeopathic Treatment

- A homeopathic combination remedy consisting of *Phytolcca* 200c, *Calcarea fluorica* 200c, *Silicea* 30c, *Belladonna*30c, *Bryonia* 30c, *Arnica* 30c, *Conium* 30c and *Ipecacuanha* 30c in equal proportion given at the dose rate 10 pills four times daily until clinical resolution has shown promising results in in the management of udder edema in cows (Ram Naresh and Varshney, 2005)

References and Literature Reviewed

Aubry,E., Issautier, M-N., Champomier,D. and Terzan,L. (2013) Early udder inflammation in dairy cows treated by a homeopathic medicine (Dolisovet): a prospective observational pilot study. Homeopathy 102(2):139-44. doi: 10.1016/j.homp.2013.02.003.

Clarke, J.H.(1902). A dictionary of pratical materia medica. homoeopathic publishing Company; 1902.

Day, C. (1986). Clinical trials in bovine mastitis – use of nosodes for prevention, The British Homoeopathic Journal 75: 11-14.

Ebert, F., Rudolf Staufenbiel, Julia Simons, Laura Pieper (2017). Randomizes, blinded controlled clinical trial shows no benefit of homeopathic mastitis treatment in dairy cows. J. Dairy Sci.100:4857-4867.

Ekert, G.(2013). Geschichtliche Entwicklung der Veterinärhomöopathie von Hahnemann bis Heute . Zeitschrift für Ganzheitliche Tiermedizin . 27: 78-81, DOI: 10.1055/s-0032-132877

Gordon, P., Kohler, S., Reist, M., van den Borne, B., Menéndez González, S. and Doherr, M.(2012). Baseline survey of health prophylaxis and management practices on Swiss dairy farms, Schweizer Archiv für Tierheilkunde. 154: 371–379, DOI: 10.1024/0036-7281/a00036.

https://dairy.ahdb.org.uk/technical-information/animal-health-welfare/mastitis/4/

https://en.wikipedia.org/wiki/Mastitis_in_dairy_cattle

Keller, D. and Sundrum,A. (2018).Comparative effectiveness of individualized homeopathy and antibiotics in the treatment of bovine clinical mastitis: randomized controlled trial. Vet.Rec. 182:407-407. https://doi.org/10.1136/vr.104555.

Klocke, P., Fidelak, C.(2010). Homöopathische Konzepte in der Euterge-sundheit, Lebendige Erde 3 : 42-45.

Klocke, P.,Ivemeyer,S., Heil, F and Walkenhorst, M. (2007). Treatment of bovine subclinical mastitis with homeopathic remedies.. 3rd QLIF Congress, Hohenheim, Germany, March 20-23, 2007Archived at http://orgprints.org./view/projects/int_confqlif 2007.html

León, L., Nürnberg, M., Andersson, R.(2006). Naturheilverfahren auf Bioland- und Demeter-Betrieben, Ökologie und Landbau. 140: 44-46.

MacLeod, G.(2012). The treatment of cattle by homoeopathy. Random House; 2012 Jun,12 Bellavite, P., Ortolani, R. and Conforti, A. (2006). Immunology and homeopathy. 3. Experimental studies on animal models. Evidence-Based Complementary and Alternative Medicine. 3:171-186.

Phatak, S.R. (2002).Materia Medica of Homoeopathic Medicines. B. Jain Publishers; 2002.

Ram Naresh and Varshney,J.P.(2005). Management of bovine udder affections with a combination homeopathic therapy. Homeopathic Links.18:104-106

Rv, Z. Complete Repertory (CR). Computer version Mac Repertory Millennium. 2000.

Schulz-Stübner, S. (2016). Geschichtliche Entwicklung und Public-Health-Aspekte, In: Multiresistente Erreger, Diagnostik – Epidemiologie – Hygiene – Antibiotika. Stewardship Schulz-Stübner, S., Dettenkofer, M., Mattner, F., Meyer, E. and Mahlberg, R. (Eds.), Springer-Verlag Berlin Heidelberg, 2016, 1-14.

Wallmann, J. (2016).Veterinary antimicrobial sales, In: Federal Office of Consumer Protection and Food Safety, Paul-Ehrlich-Gesellschaft für Chemotherapie e.V. (Ed.), Varshney,J.P. (2006). Thelitis in Dairy Animal. Homeopathic Links 19: 218.

Varshney,J.P. and Ram Naresh (2004). Evaluation of a homeopathic complex in the clinical amangement of udder diseases of riverine buffaloes. Homeopathy 93: 17-20

Varshney, J.P. and Ram naresh (2005). Comparative efficacy of homeopathic and allopathic systems of medicine in the management of clinical mastitis of Indian dairy cows. Homeopathy 94:81-85.

Varshney, J.P. and Swaminarayan, S. (2007). Research Findings. Homeopathic bioefficacy and management of Animal health.1st edn. Sintex Imetrmational limited, Kalol, Gujarat, India.

14

Therapeutic Pratice of Homeopathy in Veterinary Medicine

The practice of veterinary homoeopathy has existed since Hahnemann's time. During recent years it has emerged from the shadows and appears to be growing exponentially, expanding in many directions. Veterinary homeopathy has strongest modern tradition in Europe particularly in Germany, France and Great Britain. European Union committee has urged recently to cut the use of antimicrobials in human as well as in animals to an essential level for maintaining the effectiveness of antimicrobials and to deal with the problems of emergence of resistance among microbes.

Tradition of veterinary homeopathy is as old as humans. Initially homeopathic drugs viz. *Aconitum napellus*, *Camphora, Nux vomica* and *Opium* were used for the treatment of certain diseases of horses and cattle as early as 1833 by German Practitioner – Guillaume Lux. Since then veterinary homeopathy has progressed considerably despite the apparent difficulty in adopting the patient questioning technique, lack of expression of subjective feelings and lack of experimental data.

Despite the emphasis on individualizing a homeopathic medicine to an ailing patient by traditional homeopaths, homeopathic combinations remedies (a mixture of synergistic homeo drugs) are gaining popularity during these days owing to their broad spectrum activity and their ability to cover many clinical manifestations of a particular disease. Homeopathic drugs have been tried in the management of many diseases of farm animals (mastitis, blood in milk, thelitis, udder odema ,diarrhea, pyrexia, anestrus, retained placenta, wart, wound, anaemia etc) ,equines (warts, colic, lameness etc), pigs (still birth) and companion animals (diarrhea, fever, anaemia, babesiosis, hemorrhagic syndrome, cardiac arrhythmias, epilepsy, urinary tract diseases, hepatic disorders, etc.) with appreciable success of varying degree in India and abroad.

Whatever homeopathic treatment is being practiced in animals has been borrowed from human homeopathy. There is hardly any proving on animals. It has taken for granted that homeopathic drug have the similar effect in animals as in humans. In humans there are subjective and objective symptoms and psychological expression of thought process whereas in animals there are no subjective symptoms and thought process is different leading to absence of many expressions.

Homeopathic Veterinary Practice: Foreign scenario

Homeopathic drugs are being increasing used in animal treatment in Armenia, Belgium, Bosnia , Herzegovina, Bulgaria, Czech Republic, Finland, Germany, Greece, Ireland, Israel, Norway, Serbia, Spain, Sweden, Switzerland, United Kingdom– member countries of European council of Classical Homeopathy. Homeopathy is also used in Brazil. Animals are treated using homeopathic drugs for both acute and chronic conditions such as eczema, eye inflammation, allergies, cough; diseases of gastrointestinal tract, urinary tract, liver , thyroid, loco motor system, nervous system; diabetes; hormonal disturbances; injuries and behavioral problems. A legislation restriction has been imposed on the practice ofhomeopathy in animals in Ireland, Sweden and the United Kingdom. In Ireland and in the United Kingdom treatment of animals using homeopathy is allowed to veterinarians only. Veterinarians in Sweden are not allowed to prescribe homeopathic medicines. In Germany veterinarians are permitted to use only specifically registered homeopathic remedies in food producing animals. In Armenia and Serbia only homeopaths prescribe homeopathic remedies. In Finland and Sweden, homeopathic drugs are in the doping list (The Homeopathic Treatment of Animals in Europe, 2007). Many research studies on bovine mastitis (Day, 1986), Kennel cough (Day, 1987), rectal prolapse in pig (Searcy and Gujardo, 1994), still birth in swine (Day, 1984), post-partum anoestrus (Williamson and Others, 1995), effect of *Chelidonium* on reducing cholesterol in rabbits (Baumans and Others, 1987), anti-inflammatory effect of *Hypericum perforatum* (Varma and Others, 1988) and of *Arnica montana* in rat model (Desai and Others, 1992), labor facilitating effect of *Caulophyllum* in cows and pigs (Day, 1985), *Arsenic album* in neonatal diarrhoea (Kayne and Rafferty, 1994) have appeared in the literature.

Homeopathic Veterinary Practice: Indian scenario

Homeopathic practice in animals in India is at present in the hands of unqualified persons. The homeopathic drugs are being used in the animals by the farmers themselves, veterinarians (with no systematic knowledge of homeopathy) and other persons on the basis of drugs being used in human treatment .Individuals are making very high claims. But it remains to be proved scientifically. Whatever information on homeopathy in veterinary practice is given in this chapter has been borrowed from the information available on the internet. There is a dearth of scientific proven information on the use of homeopathic drugs in the treatment of animal diseases. That's why it is difficult to state that to what extent homeopathic treatment will be effective in diseases indicated. It appears that both single homeopathic drugs and homeopathic combination remedies have been used in different trials. Some trials on the use of homeopathic combination remedies/single homeopathic drug in the management of mammary affection/ infections in buffaloes (Varshney and Ram Naresh, 2004) and in cows (Varshney and RamNaresh, 2005, Ram Naresh and Varshney, 2005, Sharma *et al.*, 2006, Varshney, 2007, Chandel *et al.*, 2009), anoestrus in dairy animals (Kumar *et al.*, 2004, Kumar *et al.*, 2006), non specific diarrhoea in calves (Ram Naresh and Varshney, 2004), diarrhoea in pups (Varshney, 2006a), canine viral gastroenteritis (Varshney, 2006b), canine babesiosis (Chaudhuri and Varshney, 2007a), anaemia management in dogs with babesiosis (Chaudhuri and Varshney, 2007b), hypolipidaemic properties of homeocomplex (Bandyophadhyay *et al.*, 2007), cardiac arrhythmias in dogs (Varshney and Chaudhuri, 2007), haematuria in dogs (Varshney, 2013 b), epilepsy in dogs (Varshney, 2006), gall bladder diseases in canine (Bandyopadhyay *et al.*, 2010) and osteoarthritis in dogs (Varshney, 2016b) have been published in International and National journals. Studies on evaluation of homeopathic drugs in hepatopathies (in rats model and clinical cases in dogs); pyrexia syndrome (Brewer's yeast induced pyrexia in albino mice, and clinical cases in dogs); haematuria in dogs; seborrhea in dogs; stye in dogs; wounds in animals, and arrhythmias in dogs have also been conducted at Indian Veterinary Research Institute, Izatnagar (Annual Reports IVRI Izatnagar, Varshney and Swaminarayan, 2007). Calcarea carb 30c/200c has shown efficacy in relieving symptoms associated with transitional cell carcinoma in a dog (Varshney and Swaminarayan, 2018). Most of the researches on the use of homeopathic drugs in animal diseases in India suffer from small number of patients in the trial, lack of substantiation of research findings by other researchers, lack of blind and control trials and repeatability of results. Curiously published reports on the use of homeopathic drugs in animal health care has done little to convince veterinarians trained in modern medicine possibly due to inappropriate research procedures to satisfy a modern veterinarian. This necessitates further research satisfying both the basic tenets of homeopathy as well as of allopathy. Animal experimentation is a well accepted research tool in modern medicine. Randomized controlled clinical trials, which are lacking in most of the Indian works on homeopathy, are also bastion of modern scientific clinical trial. Unfortunately neither of these methodologies is appropriate to homeopathy. What is needed is a large scale placebo controlled clinical trial under field conditions. Wherein at least disease diagnosis is based on sound scientific footings including history, clinical manifestations, laboratory investigations, electrocardiography/ echocardiography, ultrasonography, radiography and / or endoscopy as the case may be. In homeopathy, uniqueness of the individual is the key factor for selecting the drug and its potency. Actually this factor hinders the controlled randomized large scale clinical trials. In one study, *Rhus tox* was used in the randomized group of osteoarthritis in humans and found not to have impact greater than placebo as remedy was not matched with the individuals symptoms (Shipley *et al.*1983). While *Rhus tox* when used in patients of fibromyalgia whose entire picture matched with *Rhus tox* showed significantly better results than placebo (Fischer *et al.,* 1989).

Are These Practices in Line with Modern Scientific Methodology?

Curiously published reports on the use of homeopathic drugs in animal health care has done little to convince veterinarians trained in modern medicine possibly due to inappropriate research procedures to satisfy them. This necessitates further research satisfying both the basic tenets of homeopathy as well as allopathy. Animal experimentation is a well-accepted research tool in modern medicine. Double blind, cross-over trials are also bastion of modern scientific clinical trial. Unfortunately neither of these methodologies is appropriate to homeopathy. Since homeopathy is individualized medicine where symptoms of the patients are matched with the symptoms of the drug and modern medicine is based on double blind, randomized and control trials, a compromising approach will facilitate scientific approach. What is needed is a large scale clinical trial under field conditions. Wherein at least disease diagnosis is based on sound scientific footings including history, clinical manifestations, laboratory investigations, electrocardiography, ultrasonography, radiography and / or endoscopy as the case may be.

Treatment of Animals with Homeopathy

Homeopathy has been in practice for the treatment of large animals since the beginning of the homeopathy. It is based on human homeopathy. No separate proving on animals are available. Almost all thing in the practice of homeopathy in animals have been borrowed from human homeopathy. Information available on the use of different homeopathic drugs in the treatment of different ailments in animals has been complied. Whatever information is available seems to be on personal experience of individuals rather than standard proven studies.

Practice of Homeopathy in Bovine

Diseases	Homeopathic Drugs Indicated
Actinobacillosis	Kali hydriodicum, Merc iodatus flavus, Merc iodatus ruber
Actinomycosis	

Bony Swelling	Heckla lava 1M
Ulcearation of Skin	Acid flour 30
Foot Ascess	Belladona200, Hepar sulf, Silicea
Agalactia	Ricinus com+ Urtica urens+five phos
Anthrax	Ars alb 1M, Lachesis, Echinacea
Abdominal Pain	
Indigestion & Constipation	Nux vomica 200
Bad Fodder	Arsenic album 200
Excess green	Colchicum200
Urine Retention	Cantharis200
Flatulence	Mag phos+Nux vomica
Arthritis	Broynia, Rhus tox, Arnica, Conium mac, Ferum phos
Anaplasmosis	Trinitrotoluene (TNT), Crotalus horridus, Phos, China, Phytolaca
Anoestrous	
Inactive ovaries	Iodum 30
Silent heat	Pulsatilla
Regularization of heat Cycle	Sepia 200
Delayed 1st estrus	Pulsatilla 30c daily one week
Derranged estrus cycle (ovarian cyst)	Natrum mur 30 or 200c daily upto 10 days.
Babesiosis	China offi, Ficus religiosa, Millefolium, Phos, Crotalus horridus, Pulsatilla.
Bronchitis	Aconite, Bryonia, Kali brom, Ars alb, Antim tart, Kali bich.
Bruises	Arnica, Ruta g.
Burns & Scald	
Minor	Cantharis200
Deep burns	Kali bich 200
Suppuration	Hepar sulph
Burn pain	Capsicum 200
Gangrene	Ars alb200
Botulism	
Difficult swallowing	Gelsemium 200
Fore limb paralysis	Plumbum 30
Hind limb paralysis	Conium mac 200
Fore limb muscle Stiffness	Curare 30
Paralysis of throat & mouth	Lathyrus sativum 1M
Black Quarter	Hepar sulph, Rhus tox

Trauma in Neonates	Arnica 30c frequently every 10 min. till response (during dystokia)
Shock in Neonates	Aconitum napellus
Edema and Anuria	Apis mellifica 30C (hrly till effect)
Fever	Belladonna 200c 2-3 doses every 30 minutes.
Diarhhoea (teething)	Chamomilla 30 c 6 hrly
Diarrhoea (weanlings)	Arsenic album 30c PO TID
Diarrhiea (with straining)	Mercuris corrosivus 30c PO BID
Anaemia in young ones	Ferrum metallicum 6x PO BID
Strogyles and tapeworms	Chenopodium 6x daily for 14 days.
Ketosis	Lycopodium, Senna

Practice of Homeopathy in Caprine

Diseases	**Homeopathic Drugs Indicated**
Bone Health	Calc phos 30 c at weaning
Caprine Arthritis Encephalitis	
Hind limb arthritis	Conium 30c
Staggering and falling to left	Stromonium 200 c
Cold	Carbo veg 30c
Constipation kids	Nux vomica 30c
Over eating kids	Nux vomica 30 c
Dehydration	China 30 C
Clostridial Diseases	Clostridium 30c
Demodicosis	Sulphur 30c Hepar sulph 30c (pustules)
Diarrhoea	Arsenic alb 30c
Emotional Trauma	Ignatia 30c
Enterotoxaemia	Clostridum 30c. (nosode)
Prevention	Clostridum 30c (nosode)
Mild symptoms	Pyrogenium and Arsen alb 200c
Facial Eczema	FE Nosode.
Spring eczema	Hypericum 30c
Liver problem	Chelidonium 30c
Joint ill	Bryonia 30c
Navel infections	Pyrogenium 30c
Nerve damage	Hypericum 200c
Pneumonia	
Moist cough, frothy	Ant. Tart 30c
Harsh chest sound	Bryonia 30c
Spasmodic cough	Drosera 30c

Kids Failure to Thrive	Baryta carb 30c
Scours	Rotavirus nosode.
Shock + Bruising	Arnica 30c
Shock + Trauma	Arnica / Acon / Bellis Pers
Emotional shock	Aconite
Urinary Calculi	Uri Calc.
Weakness associated with scour of difficult birth	Phos ac 30 c
Mastitis	Ipecacuanha 30c , Phytolacca 30c
Orf	Arnica 200
Infertility in male	
Under developed male with low libido	Lycopodium clavatum 200c one dose every 20 days
Excess breeding low libido	China officionalis 30c daily for 10 days
Breeding aversion from pain	Sepia 30 c weekly for one month
Retained Placenta (RP)	
Cervix relaxation	Caulophyllum 30c BID
Involution and expulsion of membranes	Pulsatilla 30c BID
Excessive bleeding with Membrane retention	Sabina 30c BID
RP with metritis	Sepia 30c BID

Practice of Homeopathy in Equine

Diseases	**Homeopathic Drugs indicated**
Abortion	Arnica, Sabina, Secale, Pulsatilla, China, Rhus tox
Bronchitis	Aconite, Bryonia, Belladona, Spongia, Ars alb, Pulsatilla.
Common cold	Aconite 200, Nux vomica 200
Short dry cough	Rhus tox 200
Cough, sneezing, Watery nasal discharge	Arsenic album 200
Difficult breathing, dry spasmodic cough	Bryonia 200
Profuse corryza with much sneezing	Merc sol.
Colic	
Bad food, cold water	Arsenic album + Aconite
Constipation, bloat	Nux vomica 200
Hard, dry, black feces	Opium200
Restlessness, ears cold	Chamomilla200
Flatulence	Colchicum200
Urine retention	Cantharis200
Dystokia	Arnica + Caulophyllum

Fatigue	
Fatigue after exercise	Arnica200
With loss of appetite	Nux vomica200
Bloody urine	Canabis 200
Fistula Or Sinus	
Salivary gland	Pulsatilla200
Founder	Aconite, Bryonia,Veratum alb, Rhus tox
Watery swellings or dark looking ulcers with foetid discharge	Secale cor 200
Small ulcers discharging thick matter and bleed easily	Merc vivus 200
Glanders	Ars alb, Merc sol, Sulphur

Practice of Homeopathy in Poultry

Homeopathy seems convenient in poultry because of ease of administration direct in mouth, food or in water.

Diseases	**Homeopathy Drugs Indicated**
Immunity boost in bacterial diseases	Echinacea 30c
Cold ,wet, bluish, unresponsive	Carbo veg 30c
Emotional stress	Ignatia 30c
Enlarged / Impacted crop	Nux vomica 30c
Infections	Pyrogenium 30c
Nerve damage	Hypericum 200c
Runts (failure to thrive)	Baryta carb 30c
Shock, Trauma	Arnica 30c
Soft shells	Calc phos 30 c
Sun stroke / Heat stress	Nat.mur 30c
For weight gain	Alfa alfa 30c
Bumble Foot	Arnica 30
Pneumonia	Ant. Tart 30c
Pneumonia with rattling cough	Bryonia 30c

Practice of Homeopathy in Leporine

Diseases	**Homeopathic Drugs Indicated**
Snuffles and Pneumonia	Aconite 30c (repeat hourly three doses. If no response in 12 hrs. give Bryonia 30 and phosphorus 30 alternately)
Eye problem	Arnica 30c thrice daily. Euphrasia 10% eye drops
Fleas and Ear mites	Sulphur 200 one dose weekly for three occasions
Hair balls	Occasional dose of Sulphur 30, liquid paraffin 10 ml orally

Nephritis	Aconite 30. One dose Arsenic alb 30
Wounds	Calendula cream or liquid
Pain (laceration)	Hypericum lotion externally + Hypericum 6 internally every two hours.
Tumours (MG)	Phytolacca 30. BID
Abscess	Drain+ Calendula dressing+Hepar sulph

Practice of Homeopathy in Pet birds

Diseases	**Homeopathic Drugs Indicated**
Injury, blunt trauma	Arnica
Shock, emotional trauma	Aconite
Grief following death of mate	Ignatia
Fracture	Symphytum
Stiff joints	Rhus tox
Wet, cold	Dulcamara
Cold (weather change)	Arsenicum album
Collapse	Carbo veg.
Open wound	Hypericum
Punctured wound	Ledium
Morose birds	Staphisagria
Sun stroke	Glonoinium
Feather Problems	
Damage sue to over heating in room	Sulphur
Feather plucking, bereaved, excited	Ignatia
Feather plucking, moody, broody	Sepia
Feather pluccking, boredom, itchy	Sulphur

Practice of Homeopathy in Canine

Diseases	**Homeopathic drugs Indicated**
Abscess, infection, pus	
Acute painful	Hepar sulph
Per acute, red ,hot, painful	Belladonna
Not healing but discharging	Calc. sulph
Abscess with fever	Pyrogenium
Chronic	Silica
Anal glands	Silica
Anaphylaxis	
Acute	Aconitum
Swelling on face, dry m.m	Apis mellifica
Anorexia	Ignatia, Lycopodium, Nux vomica

Arthritis	
Red, swollen joint (relief by cold Application)	Apis mellifica
Aggravate by motion, worst in warm Weather	Bryonia
Exostoses	Calc.fluor
Small joint, worst in hot weather	Ledum
Worst in cold weather	Rhus tox
Sprain	Ruta grav.
Arthritis, stiff joint, back pain, rheumatism	Rhus tox
Behavioral Disorders	
Fear	Gelsemium
Panic	Aconite
Panic when left alone	Arsenic album
Moroseness (depression)	Natrum mur
Excitement	Belladonna, Nux vomica
Noise phobia	Belladonna, Gelsemium, Nux vomica, Phosphorus
Sexual excitement	Gelsemium,Staphisagria
Urine spraying	Cantheris, Staphisagria
Bruising, injury, pain, inflammation, shock	Arnica
Collapse	Carbo veg
Constipation	
With straining , Vomiting on over eating, weak legs, back pain	Nux vomica
Small , knotty faeces	Nux vomica
Dry feces with much effort	Sulphur
Cystitis	
With hematuria, constant urge	Cantheris
With crystalluria	Sarsaparilla
Sudden, painful	Aconite
Dry cough bouts, joint swelling and Pain better on rest, Joint pain, swelling better on rest, irritability and constipation	Bryonia
Diarrhoea	
With vomiting, chilly feeling, blood in feces, small thirst, dry mouth	Arsenic album
Wet mouth , thirsty, chilly	Mercurius solubilus
Variable consistency	Pulsatilla
Worst in morning	Sulphur
Ear Diseases	
Pinna red, hot, painful	Belladonna

Watery,yellow discharge	Calc.sulph
Weeping,smelly discharge	Graphites
Purulent discharge	Hepar sulph
Purulent discharge with foul smell	Mercurius solubilus
Not smelly, not itchy	Sulphur
Aural hematoma	Arnica, Hamammelis
Eye Problems	
Thick, sticky, yellow discharge	Euphrasia
Corneal Ulcers	Mercurius corrosivus
Chronic ulcer	Conium
Conjunctivitis from cold wind	Aconitum, Euphrasia
Conjunctivitis due to sun light	Mercurius solubilus
Purulent (greenish yellow discharge)	Pulsatilla
Entropion	Rhus tox
Corneal injury	Ledum
Eczema , dermatitis, scalds, burns	Cantheris
Dental plague (cure and prevention)	Fragaria
False pregnancy	
Submissive behavior	Pulsatilla
Bad tempered ,moody	Sepia
With milk secretion	Urtica low potency
Fracture healing, repair of joint cartilage, ligament, tendon, corneal ulcers	Symphytum
Heart Problems	
Supporting heart	Digitalis low potency
Cardiac insufficiency	Crataegus
With congestive cough	Apongia
Heat Stroke	
Dramatic symptoms	Aconitum
Exhaustion and stupor	Glonoinium
Mange, flea allergy, dermatitis, itching, scratching, dandruff, scabs sores, greasy skin	Sulphur
Prostate hyperplasia	Thuja
Pyometra	Sepia
Ringworm	Bacillinum, Sepia, Kali arsenicum
Seborrhoea	Sulphur, Kali sulphuricum Natrum muriaticum, Arsenic
Skin Diseases	
Urticarial rashes	Apis mell., Urtica

Hair loss, chilly personality	Arsenicum
Sticky discharge	Graphites
Pyoderma (purulent discharge)	Hepar sulph, Mercurius corrosivus
Superficial dermatitis	Sulphur
Sprain, tendon problems. Injuries to bone	Ruta grav.
Transmisible veneral granuloma	Thuja
Urinary incontinence Senior dogs	Causticum
Vomiting, retching/nausea, thirst for small quantity of water (vomited immediately) iching, erythema, flaking, anxiety, restlessness, diarrhoea	Arsenic album
Vomiting after drinking large amount of water, Jaundice, hemorrhage, fear of thunder, Nerve weakness of hind limbs and fear of fire crackers	Phosphorus

Practice of Homeopathy in Feline

Diseases	**Homeopathic Drugs Indicated**
Digestive problems on spoiled food or on over feeding	Nux vomica
Hair balls	
Hair balls with stomach upsets, or alternating constipation and diarrhea.	Nux vomica, Pulsatilla
Cough cold (exposure to Extreme temperature)	Aconitum napellus
Influenza (early stage)	Aconite
Sneezing	
worst from cold with runny eyes and nose	Arsenic album, Natrum mur
Asthma, bronchitis	Phosphorus.
Dry, itchy, scaly skin (flea dermatitis)	Arsenicum Album
Abscess, infection, inflammation	Hepar Sulph
Alopecia	Arsenic ablum, Nat.mur
Feline Urological Syndrome	
Cystitis with hematuria, frequent painful urination	Cantheris
Crystals	Hydrangea
Kidney stones or obstruction in urinary tract	Berberis vulgaris
Separation anxiety, fear of loud noise	Calcarea carbonica
Joint Pain and Arthritis	Rhus toxicodendron
Pain, inflammation, injury	Arnica montana.

Practice of Homeopathy in Chelonian (Turtle/Tortoise)

Diseases	**Homeopathic Drugs Indicated**
Post-hibernation lethargy and anorexia	Camphora 30c.
Anorexia	Alfa alfa Q
Mouth rot	
Ulceration and necrosis	Calcarea fluorica
Yellow, thick, lumpy discharge	Calcarea sulphurica
Suppuration	Silicia
Nasal discharges	
Thin watery discharge	Arsenic album
Yellow offensive and corrosive	Acid nitricum
Corneal ulcer	Acid nitricum
Egg binding	Sepia 30c.

Common Homeopathic Drugs and Their Characteristics

Arnica –It is a valuable drug in cases of injuries both physical and mental. It has potential to reduce bruishing ,pain, shock and hemorrhage.

Aconitum- It is a drug of choice for mental shock, panic or any other very sudden disturbance of equilibrium.

Hypericum – It is a drug usually recommended in cases of injury in areas rich in nerve-endings (e.g. feet and tail).

*Led*um - It is prescribed in cases of puncture wounds.

Calendula lotion – It is recommended for wound management because of its healing , antiseptic effects, and soothing properties.

Hepar sulph- It is considered as homeopathic antibiotic and indicated in cellulitis, acute septic infection.

Silica – It is recommended in chronic suppuration.

Natrum sulphuricum – A good medicine where there is cranial injury and concussion,

*Symphytu*m – A good choice in cases of fractures or bone injury.

Ruta – It is a drug used in cases of damage of ligament (fibrous) or periosteum.

Rhus toxicodendron - It is used in cases of muscle injury.

References and Literature Reviewed

Animals &Homeopathy Info [Internet]. Slideshare.net. 2018 [cited 13 May 2018];Available from:https://www.slideshare.net/OwenHomeopathics1/animals-Homeopathy info?from_m%20_app=android

Bandyopadhyay,S. , Varshney,J.P. and Ghosh, M.K. (2007). Evaluation of hypolipidemic and hepatoprotective efficacy of a homeopathic complex in mice fed on cholesterol enriched diet. Indian J.Vet.Med.27:142-143.

Bandyopathyay, S., Varshney,J.P., Hoque,H., Swarup,D., Biswas, T.K., Bora, M. and Ghosh,M.K.(2010).Homeopathic treatment of cholecystitis disorders in dogs. Indian Vet.J. 2010 ; 981-983.

Baumans, V. and Others (1987). Does Chelodium 3 x lower serum cholesterol ? Br.Homeopathic J. 76:14

Chandel, B.S., Dadawala, A.I., Chauhan, H.C.Parsani,H.R. and Pankajkumar (2009). Efficacy of a Homeopathic complex and antibiotics in treatment of clinical mastitic cattle in North Gujarat. Vet. World 2:383-384.

Chaudhuri,S, and Varshney,J.P.(2007a). Clinical mangement of babesiosis in dogs with homeopathic *Crotalus horridus* 200c. Homeopathy 96:90-94.

Chaudhuri ,S. and Varshney,J.P.(2007b).Clinical management of anaemia associated with babesiosis in dogs with *Trinitrotoluenum* 200c. Homeopathic Links Autumn 20:162-164. @ Sonntag Verlog in MVS,Medizinverlage GmbH & Co. KG

Day, C. (1984). Control of stilbirths in pigs using Homeopathy. Vet.Rec.114:216.

Day, C, (1985). Dystocia prevention, Proceedings of LMHI congress,lyon Frnace.

Day, C. (1986). Clinical trials in bovine mastitis – use of nosodes for prevention, The British Homoeopathic Journal 75: 11-14.

Day, C.(1987). Isopathic prevention of kennel cough. Int. J. Vet.Homeopathy.2:57.

Day, C.(2002). Homeopathy – First Aid for Pets" (ISBN 0 9520071 0 X).

Day, C.(2002). The Homeopathic Treatment of Small Animals — Principles & Practice" (ISBN85207 216 3), February 2002

Day, C. (2002). Homeopathy for Cage and Aviary Birds. An Introduction to Homeopathy for Cage and Aviary Birds. Summer 2002 http://www.alternativevet.org

Desai, V. and Others (1992). Anti-inflammatory activity of Arnica on carragenen induced rat paw edema. 3rd IAVH Congress , Munster, 1992.

Emerging Role of Homeopathy in Animal Husbandry: An Overview by veterinary doctors |Homeopathy Resource by Homeobook.com [Internet]. Homeobook.com. 2018 [cited ay 2018];Available from:https://www.homeobook.com/emerging-role-of Homeopathy-in-animal husbandry-an-overview-by-veterinary-doctors/

Fisher, P and Others(1989). Effect of homeopathic treatment on fibrositis. Br.Med.J.299:365.

Kayne,S. and Rafferty,A. (1994). The use of Arsenic album 30 c to complement conventional treatment of neonatal diarrhea (scour) in calves. Br. Homeopathic J.83:202.

Raj Kumar, R.,Srivastava,S.K., Yadav,M.C., Harendra Kumar, Varshney ,V.P.and Varshney, J.P. (2004).Effect of homeopathic combination remedy on estrus induction and hormonal profile in anestrus cows. XX Annual Convention of ISSAR and National Symposium, Durg, 14th –16th Dec.,2004, pp 39-40.

Raj Kumar, R., Srivastava, S.K., Yadav, M.C., Varshney,V.P., Varshney,J.P. andKumar,H. (2006).Effect of a Homeopathic complex on oestrus induction and

Ram Naresh and Varshney,J.P.(2005). Management of bovine udder affections with a combination homeopathic therapy. Homeopathic Links.18:104-106

Ruddock, E. and Lade, G.(1879).The pocket manual of homeopathic veterinary medicine. London: The Homeopathic Publishing Company; 1879.

Rush, J. (2007).The handbook to veterinary homeopathy.New Delhi:B. Jain Publishers; 2007.

Searcy, R. and Guajardo, G. (1994). Three p[apers on homeopathic research. Proceedings of the American Holistic Veterinary Medical Association Annual Conference p 93.

Sharma, A.,Dhingra,P.,Pender,B.L., and Kumar.R. (2006).Bovine subclinical mastitis: prevalence and treatment with homeopathic medicine.Int.J.Cow Sci.2:40-44.

Shipley,M. and Others (1983). Controlled trial of homeopathic treatment of osteoarthritis. Lancet 1:97.

Swayne, D. and Glisson, J. (2013).Diseases of poultry. Ames, Iowa: Wiley-Blackwell; 2013.

Thakor, P.S. (2018) [Internet]. Drthakoridealcure.com. 2018 [cited 13 May 2018]; Available from: http://drthakoridealcure.com/

Varma, P. N.,Kumar, S.,Lohar,D.R., Chaturvedi,D. and Gaur,G.D. (1988). A chemo-pharmacologicalk study of *Hypericum perforatum*. Br.Homeopathic J.77:27.

Varshney,J.P. and Ram Naresh (2004). Evaluation of a homeopathic complex in the clinical amangement of udder diseases of riverine buffaloes. Homeopathy 93: 17-20

Varshney, J.P. and Ram naresh (2005). Comparative efficacy of homeopathic and allopathic systems of medicine in the management of clinical mastitis of Indian dairy cows. Homeopathy 94:81-85.

Varshney, J.P.(2006 a). Thelitis in Dairy Animals. Homeopathic Links .International Journal of Classical Homeopathy Winter 19:218 @ Sonntag Verlog in MVS,Medizinverlage GmbH & Co. KG

Varshney, J.P. (2006 b). Arsenic album in gastroenteritis in pups. Am.J.Homeopathic Medicine (Winter Issue) 99(4):296-297.

Varshney, J.P. (2006 c). Clinical management of idiopathic epilepsy in dogs with homeopathic Belladonna 200C; a case series . Homeopathy 96: 46-48.

Varshney, J.P.(2007d). Clinical Management of Acute Mastitis in Bitches with a Homeo-Complex. In: Research Findings. Homeopathic Bioefficacy and Management of Animal Health. Varshney, J.P. and Swaminarayan, S (eds). Sintex International Limited, Kalol, pp.55-59.

Vatshney,J.P.(2007e). Hepatoprotective Efficacy of A Homeopathic Combination Remedy in Phenobarbital Induced Hepatopathy in Epileptic Dogs). In: Research Findings. Homeopathic Bioefficacy and Management of Animal Health. Varshney, J.P. and Swaminarayan, S (eds). Sintex International Limited, Kalol, pp.25-28.

Varshney, J.P. (2007f) .Clinical Management of Haematuria with Uva ursi. In: Research Findings. Homeopathic Bioefficacy and Management of Animal Health. Varshney, J.P. and Swaminarayan, S (eds). Sintex International Limited, Kalol, pp.101-102.

Varshney, J.P.(2007g). Clinical Management of Haematuria with a Homeopathic-complex in a Spitz Dog. In: Research Findings. Homeopathic Bioefficacy and Management of Animal Health. Varshney, J.P. andSwaminarayan, S (eds). Sintex International Limited, Kalol, pp.103-105.

Varshney, J.P. (2007h) . A preliminary trial of a homeopathic shampoo in the management of Seborrhoea in Dogs. In: Research Findings.Homeopathic Bioefficacy and Management of Animal Health. Varshney, J.P. and Swaminarayan, S (eds). Sintex International Limited, Kalol, pp 125-127.

Varshney, J.P. (2007 i). Clinical management of cystitis in dogs with Cantheris. In: Research Findings. Homeopathic Bioefficacy and Management of Animal Health. Varshney, J.P. and Swaminarayan, S (eds). Sintex nternational Limited, Kalol, pp 106-109..

Varshney, J.P. and Chaudhuri, S. (2007). Atrial paroxysmal tachycardia in dogs andits management with homeopathic digitalis.- Two case report. Homeopathy 96 (4) :270-272.

VarshneJ.P., Deshmukh ,V.V.and Chaudhary,P.S. (2007). Clinical Management of common cold in a Labrador pup with Allium cepa 30C.. 15th All India Homeopathic Scientific Seminar, Rajkot, 21-23rd Dec.,2007.

Varshney, J.P. and Paliwal, O.P. (2007).Clinical Management of Squamous Metaplasia with Thuja in a Dog. In: Research Findings. Homeopathic Bioefficacy and Management of Animal Health. Varshney, J.P. and Swaminarayan, S (eds). Sintex InternationalLimited, Kalol, pp.148-149.

Varshney,J.P., Tandon, S.K. and Dudhgaonkar (2007).Anti-inflammatory Activity of a Homeo-complex in Carrageenan Induced Hindpaw Odema in Rats. In: Research Findings. Homeopathic Bioefficacy and Management of Animal Health. Varshney, J.P. and Swaminarayan, S. (eds). Sintex International Limited, Kalol, pp.29-33.

Varshney,J.P., Tandon,S.K. and Bhat, A.S. (2007).Evaluation of Anti-pyretic Efficacy of Homeopathic Drugs in Brewer's Yeast Induced Pyrexia.In: Research Findings. Homeopathic Bioefficacy and Management of Animal Health. Varshney, J.P. and Swaminarayan, S. (eds). Sintex International Limited, Kalol, pp.96-10.

Varshney,J.P., Paliwal, O.P. and Hoque, M. (2007).Use of A Homeo-complex as An Adjunct Therapy in the Management of Infectious Canine Hepatitis. In: Research Findings. Homeopathic Bioefficacy and Management of Animal Health. Varshney, J.P. and Swaminarayan, S (eds). Sintex International Limited, Kalol, pp.60-63.

Varshney, J.P. and Swaminarayan, S. (2007). Research Findings. Homeopathic bioefficacy and management of Animal health.1st edn. Sintex Imetrmational limited, Kalol,Gujarat, India.

Varshney,J.P.and Swaminarayan, S.(2010) . Homeopathic drugs in the management of anaemia in animals. Brain Storming Session at CFTRI , Mysore

Varshney, J.P. and Swaminarayan,S, (2010). Clinical management of gastroenteritis with Arsenic album 30C in animals. XXII National Congress ofIndian Institute of Homeopathic Physicians, Delhi State Branch, Delhi

Varshney, J.P. (2011).An overview of Research in Homeopathic Veterinary Medicine in India. Liga 2011

Varshney, J.P.(2011).Diagnosis and Management of Atrial Paroxysmal Tachycardia in Dogs with Homeopathic Digitalis. Liga 2011

Varshney, J.P. and Swaminarayan, S. (2011) Clinical Management of Thelitis with homeopathic drugs in cows and buffaloes. Liga 2011.

Varshney, J.P. nd Swaminarayan, S.(2011). Clinical Management of Gastroenteritis with Arsenic album 30C in animals Asian Conference held at Ceylon.

Varshney, J.P. (2013). Clinical management of haematuric dogs with *Cantheris* 30C.Journal of Case Studies in Homeopathy.1 (2):2-6.

Varshney , J.P.(2016). Management of Osteoarthritis in dogs using a homeopathic combination remedy. Indian.J. Vet.Med. 36:148-150..

Varshney,J.P. and Swaminarayan,S. (2018). Case Study: Canine Bladder Tumour (Transitional Cell Carcinoma). 3rd International Conference onIntegrative Oncology. Nashik (19-21 Jan, 2018).

Veterinary Research – The Faculty of Homeopathy [Internet]. The Faculty of Homeopathy. 2018 [cited 13 May 2018];Available from: https://facultyofhomeopathy.org/research/veterinary-research/

Williamson, A.V. and Others (1995). A trial of Sepia 200. Br.Homeopathic J.84: 14.

15

Preventive Veterinary Homeopathy Scope and Overview

Preventive Homeopathy

Homeopathy is entirely a unique philosophy different from that of conventional modern medicine. It is considered as a tailor made system of therapy administering a medicine fitting well in the totality of physical and psychological symptoms seen in an ailing individual whether it is human or animal. Homeopathy does not restrict to restoring health of ailing subjects (treatment of clinical diseases) but also offers scope for preventing diseases as well. It can play significant role in preventing enzootic and epizootic infectious diseases through administration of nosodes.

Nosodes

Nosodes are important class of homeopathic drugs specifically prepared from secretions or fluids of the diseased subjects or their infectious agents in the similar manner as other homeopathic drugs are made (process of dilution and succession). The word "nosode " is derived from the Greek "nosos" (disease) and "eidos" (like). Nosodes are potentized remedies prepared from diseased tissues , discharges (products of disease) or disease causing agents (bacteria or virus) in a specialized manner following standard protocol. Dr. Samuel Hahnemann first prepared remedies from diseased tissues (mainly the miasmatic nosodes) for the three miasms (Psora, Sycosis and Syphilis) corresponding as Psorinum, Medorrhinum, and Syphylinum. Of which first two have common use in veterinary homeopathy. The nosodes have undergone proving similar to other drugs, and their use in veterinary homeopathy is in the same manner as with any other remedy i.e. matching patient symptoms with those of the remedy.

Nosodes for Disease Prevention

Later in the 1800s, the use of nosodes developed for specific diseases started , such as anthrax in cattle (Anthracinum), and distemper in dogs (Distemperinum).Later on a nosode Hydrophobinum (30c potency) was developed from the saliva of the rabid dog by Dr. Constantine Hering to treat and prevent rabies in dogs and humans. Now a days this nosode is known as “Lyssin”. Heart worm and Parvo nosodes claimed to offer some promise to boost immunity. These medicines are not antibiotics and do not possess bactericidal or bacteriostatic activity (Banerjee, 2006). Examples of nosodes prepared and used in humans are Baccilinum (from tuberculous sputum), Medorrhinum (from gonorrhea agent), Carcinosin (from cancerous tissues); Psorinum (psoric preparation), Pyrogenium (infected pus), Syphilinum (syphilitic germs’ preparation), Tuberculinum (pus of tubercular), Typhoidinum (*Salmonella typhi’* preparation), Variolinum (smallpox eruptions’ preparation), Ambra grisea (whale), Aviare (tuberculin of chicken), Anthracinum (anthrax poison from spleen of affected cattle or sheep), Mallandrinum (grease in horse), Hydrophobinum or lyssin (saliva of a rabid dog), Secale cor (fungus growing on the seeds of the secale cerale), and *Ustilago maydis* (fungus, growing on the stem of Indian corn).

The recorded use of nosode in animals dates back to 1831 when Wilheim Lux used 30 CH dilution of a drop of mucus from glander affected animal (AAHP and AHVMA,1991). Nosodes have also been used in Livestock (Day,1995, Macleod, 1981,1991. 1994). Day (1986) and Klocke and Fidelak (2010) evaluated nosodes for mastitis control. Day (1986) evaluated a combined nosode of five pathogens keeping a placebo control. 25% of the placebo controlled animals and 2.5% of the nosode treated animals developed mastitis. The homeopathic treated cows had a lower average somatic cell count per month of 160,000 cell counts/ml .Though , study showed encouraging results, this method of comparison made the validity of the study more difficult. In another study homeopathy was compared to internal teat sealer (Klocke and Fidelak ,2010) . The result did not showed significant difference between cows treated with homeopathy or with internal teat sealer.

Nosodes have been tried for kennel cough, distemper, hepatitis and parvo in dogs, for influenza, enteritis, feline leukemia virus and feline infectious peritonitis in cats; and influenza and herpes in horses (Day,1998).

Dr. Day initially tried nosodes in prevention of a few animal diseases. The method of preventing diseases via nosode is not yet recognized by regulatory bodies in cases where vaccination is mandatory. He successfully tried *Caulophyllum* 30c in a breeding unit of sows and obsereved significant drop in still birth rate in pigs. He also used nosode for canine tracheobronchitis (Day,1986). He prepared anud used many nosodes on his own animals, equine, feline, canine without any ill effect. He successfully used *Caulophyllum* 30c in cows to relieve calving difficulties (Day, 1995).

For the purpose of disease prevention, 30c potency of the homeopathic nosodes is usually used. Regimens and dose schedules has varied in different recommendations. Administration of nosodes for preventive purpose is usually oral. In earlier trial for kennel cough, distemper, canine hepatitis and parvo in dogs; for influenza, enteritis, feline leukemia virus, feline immunodeficiency virus, feline infectious peritonitis in cats; and influenza and herpes in horses, nosodes have been used as twice daily for 3days; followed by twice weekly for 3 weeks; followed by once monthly for 6 months; followed by a dose morning and night every 6 months (Day, 1998).

Scope of Nosodes

In India, scientific work on nosodes in the prevention of animal diseases is utterly lacking. Not a single authenticated scientific report on the use of a nosode for disease control or prevention in animals in India could be traced in Indian or foreign literature. The subject of using nosode in disease prevention and replacing vaccination with nosode is still under debate and requires more authenticated scientific trials. At present it cannot be stated with certainty that nosodes can replace vaccination or can have great role in controlling infectious diseases as scientific data is utterly lacking. Nevertheless in view of encouraging results of the trials done earlier abroad, it seems more scientific large scale controlled double blind studies are the need of the hour to provide evidence whether homeopathic nosodes can have any beneficial role in preventing infectious diseases in veterinary practice. This is a huge scientific task and needs legalization and regulation involving Veterinary council of India, Drug controller, state and central governments and academic institutions.

Prevention of Diseases by Homeopathic Drugs Other than Nosodes

Diseases at parturition as a result of physical trauma (damage occurring during difficult birth). surgical shock, side effects of anesthesia and bowing of bones can be prevented by the oral homeopathic drugs (Madrewar and Glencross, 2010). Problem associated with difficult birth can be protected by the preventive use of *Caulophyllum, Pulsatilla, Calcarea phos*. These medicines are also curative in this condition. *Arnica montana*, *Calcarea fluor* and *Straphisagria* can be used to prevent operative or post-operative shock. Rickets (bending of long bones) can be prevented by *Calcarea carbonica*, *Calcarea ph*os and *Magnesia ph*os. Post wound scars can be avoided by *Thuja* or *Silicea* (Madrewar and Glencross,2010). These are the other areas where homeopathic drugs can be used orally to prevent the illness.

References and Literature Reviewed

American Association of Homeopathic Pharmacists and the American Holistic Veterinary Medical Association. (1991). The place of homeopathic remedies in veterinary medicine., 1991, The Associations.

Banerjee, D.(2006). Augmented Textbook of Homoeopathic Pharmacy: B. Jain Publishers (P) Ltd, 2006

Day, C. (1986).Clinical trials in bovine mastitis – use of nosodes for prevention, The British Homoeopathic Journal, 1986, 75, 11-14.

Day, C. (1995).Homeopathic treatment of beef and dairy cattle, Beaconsfield, England, Beaconsfield Publisher.

Day, C. (1998). Veterinary Homeopathy: Principles and Practice. In: Complementary and Alternative Veterinary Medicine. Principles and Practice. Schoen, A.M. and Wynn, S.G. (eds). Mosby, St Louis, baltomore, Boston, Carlsbad, Chicago, Naples, NewYork, Philadelphia, Portland, London, Madrid, Mexico City, Sigapore, Sydney, Tokyo, Toronto, Wiesbaden.pp 485-513.

Klocke, P. and Fidelak C. (2010). Homöopathische Konzepte in der Eutergesundheit, Lebendige Erde 3, 2010, 42-45.

Macleod, G. (1981).The treatment of cattle by homeopathy. Saffron Walden, England, 1981, C.V. Daniel.

Macleod, G. (1991). Goats: Homeopathic remedies. Saffron Walden, England, 1991, C.V. Daniel.

Macleod, G. (1994).A veterinary materia media. Saffron Walden, England, 1994, C.V. Daniel.

Madrewar, B.O. and Glencross, M. (2010). Therapeutics of Veterinary Homeopathy and repertory.2nd edn 5th Impression. B.Jain Publishers (P) Ltd., New delhi.

16

Research in Veterinary Homeopathy

In India there are many scattered case reports on the use of homeopathic drugs in the treatment of certain ailments in animals with individual claims but these reports suffer from lack of evidence, repeatability, documentation and scientific fervor. During last 2-3 decades some reports on the evaluation of homeopathic medicines in the management of animal diseases have appeared in the literature as well as in professional seminars and conferences in India. The abstract summary of these works are given in this chapter.

Clinical Studies

Clinical Management of Udder Diseases of Riverine Buffaloes With A Homeopathic Complex

J.P. Varshney and Ram Naresh (2004)

An uncontrolled observational study was undertaken to evaluate the effectiveness of a homeopathic complex in the management of clinical udder health problems of riverine buffaloes. Cases of subclinical mastitis were excluded from the study. A total of 102 mastitic quarters (fibrosed – 40, nonfibrosed – 62) and five cases each of blood in milk and udder oedema in lactating buffaloes were treated with a homeopathic complex consisting of *Phytolacca* 200C, *Calcarea fluorica* 200C, *Silicia* 30C, *Belladonna* 30C, *Bryonia* 30C, *Arnica* 30C, *Conium* 30C and *Ipecacuanha* 30C. The diagnosis of udder diseases and recovery criterion was based on physical examination of udder and milk and CMT/WST score. Bacteriological analysis and somatic cell count were not performed.Treatment was 80 and 96.72% effective in cases of fibrotic mastitis and non-fibrosed mastitis respectively. Recovery period was 21-42 days (fibrosed) and 4-15 days (non-fibrosed). Udder oedema and blood in milk responded favourably in 2-5 days. Cost of treatment was US$ 0.07 per day. The homeopathic complex medicine may be effective and economical in the management of udder health problems of buffaloes. Definitive conclusions are premature due to the limited number of observations and lack of control group.

Clinical Management Of Bovine Udder Affections With A Homeopathic Combination Therapy

Ram Naresh and J.P. Varshney (2005)

The present clinical trial was undertaken to evaluate the efficacy of a homeopathic combination therapy in udder affections of dairy cows. Twenty-five mastitic quarters (10 fibrosed and 15 non fibrosed) and four cases of udder oedema in crossbred dairy cows (Fig.5) formed the material for present clinical trial. A homeopathic formulation consisting of *Phytolacca* 200C, *Calcarea fluorica* 200C, *Silicia* 30C, *Belladonna* 30C, *Bryonia* 30C, *Arnica* 30C and *Ipecacuahna* 30C, was given orally at the dose rate of 15 pills, twice daily, to cows affected with mastitis or udder oedema, till clinical recovery or drying off the quarter (un-recovered) supported by California mastitis test (CMT) score and physical changes of milk and udder. Twenty five quarters of clinical mastitis (nonfibrosed) treated with conventional treatment (Standard intra mammary infusion of antibiotics) were also included in the study for comparison. Results of clinical trial indicated that in fibrosed, nonfibrosed quarters and udder oedema the homeopathic combination was 70, 93.33 and 100% effective respectively. However, duration of therapy varied from 8-51 days for fibrosed mastitis and 3-32 days of nonfibrosed mastitis and 8-23 days for udder oedema. Though the efficacy of conventional treatment (intra-mammary antibiotic infusion) was lower (68%) but the average duration of treatment was quite low (5-6 days) in cases of nonfibrosed mastitis. The seven of ten fibrosed and hopeless quarters cured with above remedy with normal secretion of milk with a longer duration therapy may be very much encouraging for homeopaths to go for a large clinical trial for such conditions. However, in case of udder oedema data are scanty to draw any conclusion.

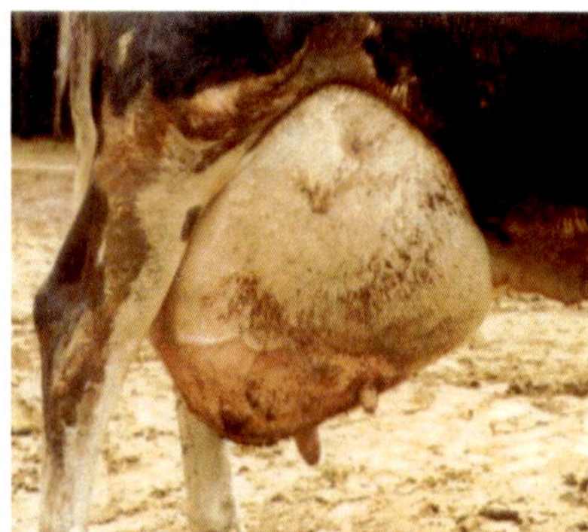

A. Fibrosed mastitis in a Holstein cow

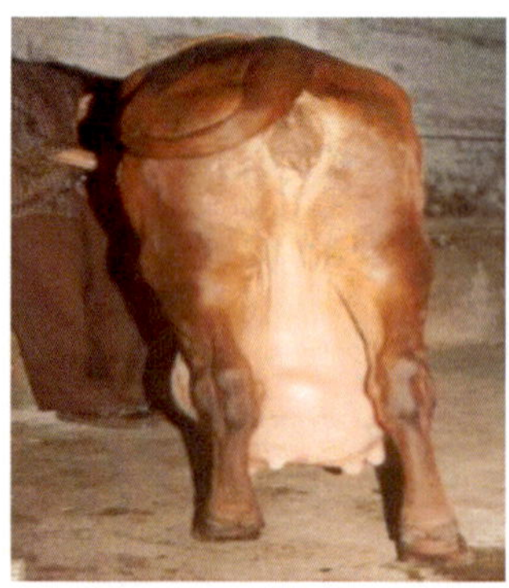

B. Udder edema in a cow

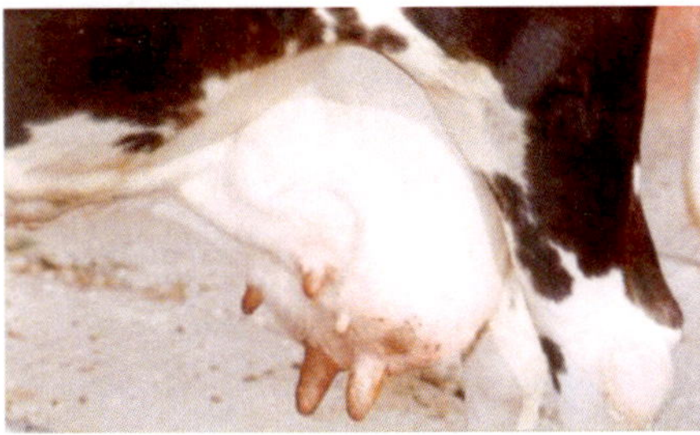

C. Holstein Frisien crossbred cow showing non –fibrosed mastitis (before treatment)

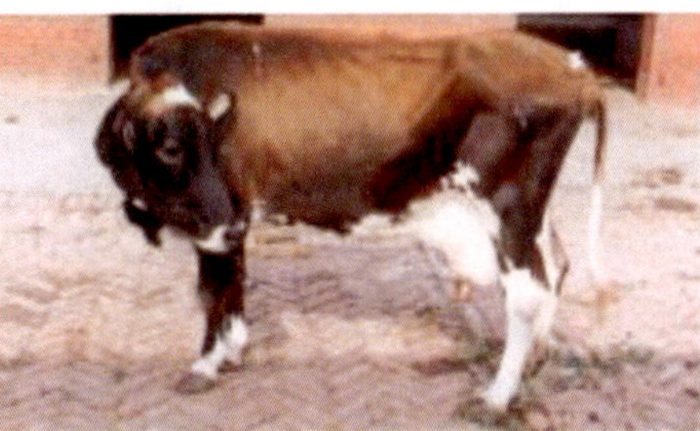

D.Cow at C after Homeopathic treatment

Fig.5. Cows showing fibrosed mastitis at A, udder edema at B, non-fibrosed mastitic cow at C and cow at (C) recovered with homeopathic treatment at D.

Comparative Efficacy of Homeopathic and Allopathic Systems of Medicine in the Management of Clinical Mastitis of Indian Dairy Cows

J.P. Varshney and Ram Naresh (2005)

The present investigation reports the treatment economics of homeopathic drugs Vs allopathic drugs in the management of mastitis. A total number of 96 mastitic quarters (nonfibrosed 67 and fibrosed 29) were treated with a homeopathic combination remedy (*Phytolacca* 200C, *Calcarea fluorica* 200C, *Silicia* 30C, *Belladonna* 30C, *Bryonia* 30C, *Arnica* 30C and *Ipecacuahna* 30C) at the dose rate of 15 pills twice daily . Another 96 quarters with acute mastitis (non-fibrosed) treated with different antibiotics were also included in the study for comparison of the systems of medicine (homeopathy vs. allopathy). The animals were selected from dairy farm of the Indian Veterinary Research Institute and also from private dairy farm. The overall efficacy of homeopathic combination remedy in the treatment of acute non fibrosed mastitis was recorded as 86.56% with a mean recovery period of 7.68±0.59 days, though recovery period varied from 3-28 days, and total cost of therapy as Rs. 21.44. Whereas quarter cure rate of antibiotic group was 59.18% with a mean recovery period of 4.54±0.20 days (range 2-15 days) and an average treatment cost of Rs. 149.20. The combination of *Phytolacca, Calc. Flour., Silicia, Belladonna, Bryonia, Arnica, Conium and Ipecac* was highly efficacious and economical in the management of fibrotic and non fibrotic mastitis in lactating dairy cows than that of antibiotics.

Clinical Management of Thelitis with Homeo Drugs in Cows and Buffaloes

J.P. Varshney (2006)

Thelitis is an inflammation of the teat usually associated with pain because of injury and is without alteration in milk. It is generally intractable to intramammary antibiotic therapy. Three cases of acute thelitis (Cows 2, Buffalo 1) were treated with Arnica 30 C @ 10 pills TID orally on the day of referral followed by Bryonia 30 C @ 10 pills TID orally from 2nd day onward for 2-3 days along with topical application of Bryonia cream (containing Bryonia alba Q 8% V/W in cream base) for 3 days. The recovery was uneventful within 3-4 days.

Clinical Management of Acute Mastitis in Bitches with a Homeo- Complex

J.P.Varshney (2007 a)

A clinical trial with a homeo-complex in the management of canine mastitis was undertaken. Ten clinical cases of mastitis (Fig.6 bitch showing swelling of mammary glands)were treated with a homeo-complex, consisting of *Belladonna 30C, Bryonia 30C, Arnica 30 C, Phytolacca 200C, Calcarea fluorica 200C, Silicia 30C, Conium 30C and Ipecacuanha 30C*, @ 4 pills thrice daily for 7 days. The diagnosis of mastitis was based on physical changes in mammary glands and milk (Fig.7) ; CMT/WST score, and leukocytosis with neutrophilia. Efficacy of the homeo-complex was 80.0 per cent in the management of mastitis in bitches. Cost of the total treatment was approximately Rs. 7.00. It seems that homeo- complex was cheap and effective in the management of canine mastitis.

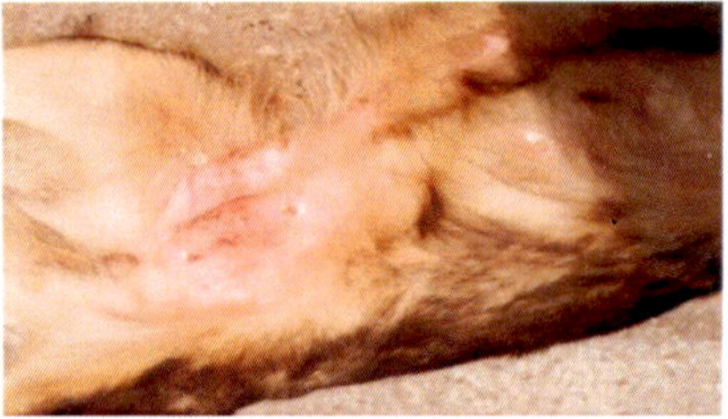

Fig. 6. Acute mastitis in a bitch showing physical changes in mammary glands

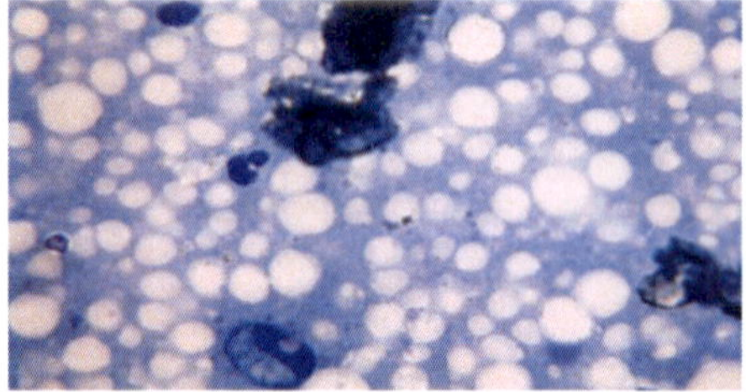

Fig. 7. Milk smear of canine mastitic milk showing the presence of neutrophils.

Hepatoprotective Efficacy of A Homeopathic Combination Remedy in Phenobarbital Induced Hepatopathy in Epileptic Dogs

J.P. Varshney (2007 b)

Epilepsy or seizure is a common neurological problem in dogs. Anticonvulsants such as phenobartital, potassium bromide, primidone, diazepam or valproic acid either alone or in combination are advocated for its management in the modern medicine. These drugs have been found as a potent inducer of hepatic enzymes leading to hepatopathy warranting discontinuance or modification of anticonvulsants in many cases. The present clinical study was undertaken to evaluate a homeopathic combination remedy for its hepatoprotective efficacy in epileptic dogs treated with phenobarbital.Twenty epileptic dogs (German shepherd 12, Boxer 2, Great Dane 1, Pomeranian 1 and Nondescript 4), aged 1 to 5 years, treated with phenobarbital @ 2-6 mg per Kg b.wt. PO bid were included in the present study. They were randomly assigned to group A and B each of 10 epileptic dogs. In group-B a homeopathic combination remedy (consisting of *Carduus marianus* Q 5%. *C'helidonium majus* Q 2%. *Andrographis paniculata* Q 5%, *Hydrastis canadenj'is*. Q 2%, *Taraxacu*m Q 2%, *Podophyllum peltdrum* Q 2%, *Ipecacuanha* Q 2% and *Carica* P Q 2% in syrup base) was also given @ one TSF PO tid in addition to phenobarbital. The seizure syndrome was clinically characterized by generalized tonic-clonic convulsions, lasting for 1-3 min., limb rigidity, paddling, chewing movements, salivation, involuntary urination and defecation and temporary loss of consciousness followed by disorientation and dullness. Based on clinical, haemato-biochemical, radiological, ultrasonographic and electrocardiographic observations, diagnosis of idiopathic epilepsy was arrived at. Initial mean values of ALT (group A 95.14 +10.74 U/I; group B 85.5 + 17.51 U/I) and alkaline phosphatase-SAP (group A 156.0 + 10.24 U/I; group B 143.8 +10.18 U/I) at the time of referral did not vary significantly between both groups and were well within normal limits. ALT (310.0 + 28.22 U/L) and alkaline phosphatase (418.0 + 30.05 U/I) values increased significantly (P< 0.0 I) in dogs of group-.A treated with phenobarbital alone for 8 weeks, indicating induction of liver enzymes. On the other hand there was no significant increase in the values of AL T and SAP in dogs of group-B given a homeo-complex in addition to phenobarbital indicating that the simultaneous use of homeopathic combination remedy was able to arrest phenobarbital induced enzyme induction in the liver and thus acted as a hepatoprotectant.

Use of A Homeo-complex as an Adjunct Therapy in the Management of Infectious Canine Hepatitis

J.P. Varshney, O.P. Paliwal and M. Hoque (2007)

Two cases of infectious canine hepatitis were diagnosed based on epidemiological considerations and clinical manifestations. The diagnosis was confirmed on the basis of intranuclear basophilic inclusions in corneal impression (Fig.9) smears of both and liver smear of the collapsed dog. Disease manifestations were characterized by tonsilar enlargement, pyrexia, nausea/vomiting, cervical lymphadenopathy, mild coughing, pulmonary rales, abdominal tenderness and pain, photophobia, blepharospasms, corneal opacity (Fig.8) , low voltage complexes, increased activities of ALT, SAP, gamma-GT and higher total bilirubin and death of one dog (non descript). Ultrasound examination revealed enlarged hypoechoic liver and distended gall bladder with thickened wall (Fig.10). Treatment was initiated with 5% DNS, cephalexin, metronidazole, homeocomplex (consisting of *Kalmegh, Carica P., chelidonium, Myrica and Chionanthus*) and a vitamin B complex and mineral supplements. Recovery was uneventful in the Pomeranian pup (Fig 11) with a definite lowering of serum enzyme activities (ALT, SAP and gamma GT) on day 7 post therapy indicating hepatic stimulating efficacy of the homeo-complex.

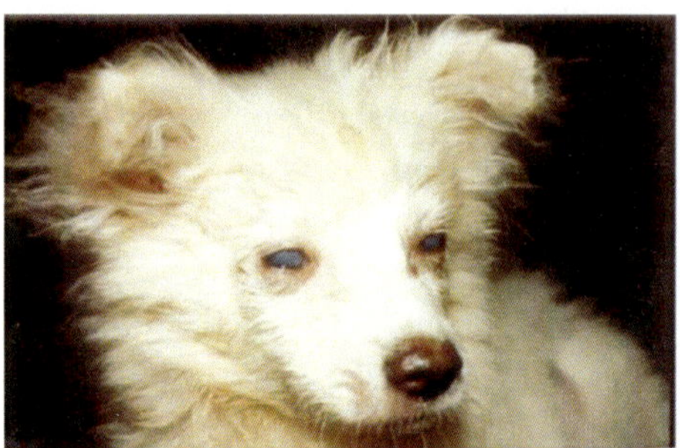

Fig. 8. Bilateral corneal odema and opacity in a Pomeranian pup suffering from infectious canine hepatitis

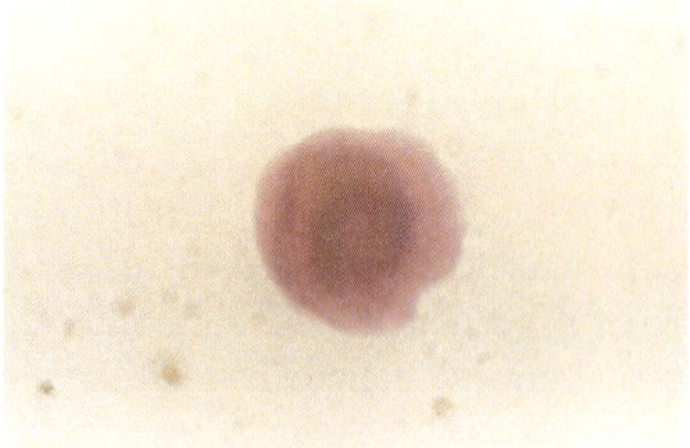

Fig. 9. Intranuclear inclusion in corneal impression smears of Pomeranian pup confirming diagnosis of infectious canine hepatitis

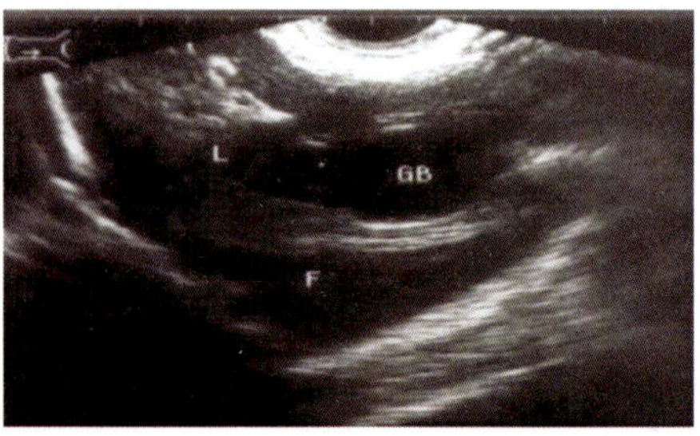

Fig. 10. Liver ultrasonogram of the treated pup with infectious canine hepatitis showing hypoechoic changes in the liver .

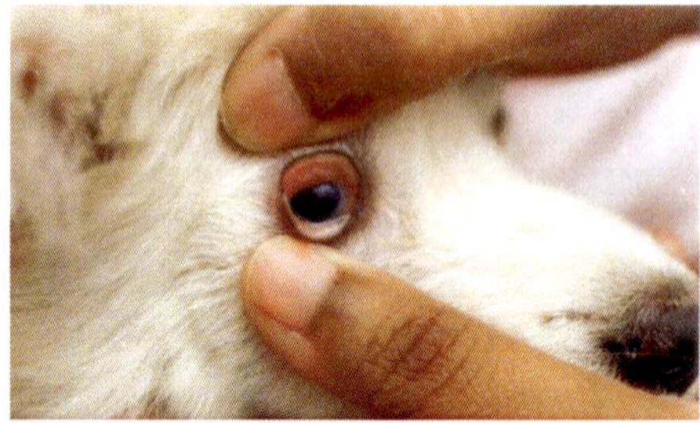

Fig.11. ICH affected Pomeranian pup with homeopathic drugs showing clearance of clouding of cornea.

Evaluation of Hepatoprotective Efficacy of a Homeo-complex in Dogs with Hepatopathy

S. Soja Saghar, J.P. Varshney and M. Hoque (2007)

The present investigation was conducted to evaluate the hepatoprotective efficacy of a homeo-complex (consisting of *Andrographis panniculata, Carica P, Chelidonium majus, Myrica ceri and Chionanthus* in syrup base as well as in pill form) in dogs with confirmed hepatopathy. 24 dogs having atleast 5 or more clinical signs of hepatopathy; a diffuse hypoechoic liver, and elevated activity of liver specific enzymes (ALT, SAP and gamma-GT), increased values of total and direct bilirubin, and lowered values of serum protein and albumin, were divided randomly into four groups of 6 dogs each (Gr. B,C,D, and E). Dogs of group B were treated with conservative therapy alone. While dogs of group C,D and E received homeo-complex in syrup base, homeocomplex in pill form and silymarin respectively in addition to conservative therapy. Another 6 apparently healthy dogs with no clinical signs, normal hepatic echotexture and normal liver specific enzyme activity served as healthy control (Gr.A) for comparison. Dogs with hepatopathy and treated with homeocomplex (group C & D) and silymarin (group E) showed faster regression of clinical signs, reduction in elevated liver specific enzyme (ALT, SAP & gamma-GT), decrease in serum total and direct bilirubin, and increase in serum total protein and albumin, and returning of normal hepatic echotexture by day 14 post therapy.

Hepatotrophic Potential of a Homeo-complex in the Management of Secondary Hepatopathy Associated with a Mixed Infection of E.canis and B.gibsoni in Dogs

Ajay Kumar and J.P.V arshney (2007)

The study was conducted to evaluate the hepatotrophic efficacy of a homeo-complex in dogs with hepatopathy associated with concurrent infection of *E.canis* and *B.gibsoni*. Ten clinical cases of concurrent infection of *E.canis* and *B.gibsoni* with confirmed hepatopathy (based on diffuse hypoechoic liver and elevated SAP 183.969±34.88 IU/L; ALT 116.69±35.42 IU/L) were treated with a homeo-complex (Consisting of *Carduus marianus, Chelidonium majus, Andrographis paniculata, Hydrastis canadensis, Taraxacum, Podophyllum, Ipecacuahana* and *Carica P*) at the rate of one teaspoonful three times daily for 14 days. The results revealed regression in clinical signs of secondary hepatic dysfunction, marked lowering of liver specific enzyme activities (SAP 44.915±22.26 U/L; ALT 50.25±10.93 U/L), decrease in serum BUN (11.4±3.26 mg/dl), and an increase in serum protein, albumin and globulin levels (6.937±0.465, 2.242±0.295, 4.493±0.400 g/dl) suggesting hepatotrophic potential of the homeopathic combination remedy in syrup form.

A Clinical Study on Antipyretic Efficacy of a Homeopathic Complex in Dogs

J.P. Varshney and Ajay Kumar (2003)

The present investigation was undertaken to evaluate antipyretic potential of a homeopathic complex in dogs. One hundred and seventy six dogs, referred at Referral Veterinary Polyclinic of the Institute during December 2001 to December 2003, were included in the present study. Of these 15, 15, 15 and 129 dogs were assigned to group A, B, C and D respectively. Dogs of group-A with a mean rectal temperature as 38.2 ± 0.10°C served as healthy control. While dogs with rectal temperature > 39°C with systemic signs were diagnosed with fever and subdivided into B, C and D groups. Dogs of group B were assigned to antipyretic treatment only after confirming their rectal temperature again at 1h. While, dogs of group C and D were treated with paracetamol (125-250 mg orally thrice daily] or a homeopathic complex consisting of *Aconite* 30 C, *Ferrum phos* 30 C, *Belladonna* 30 C, *Arsenic al*b. 30 C and *Kali mur* 30 C in equal proportions (4 pills orally at 15 min interval for 3 occasions and then four times a day) respectively. Initial diagnosis of fever was based on elevated rectal temperature (>39°C) with systemic signs. On the basis of clinical and laboratory investigations the etiology of the fever in these dogs of group B, C and D varied from infections (*Babesia gibsoni*, *B. canis*, *Ehrilchia canis*, *E. platys*, granulocytic ehrlichiosis, *Trypanosoma evansi*, concurrent infection of *Babesia* and *Ehrlichia*), cirrhosis, status epilepticus, metritis (*Escherichia coli*), cystitis (*E. coli*), mastitis (*E. coli*) and distemper. Changes in rectal temperature were recorded at 0h, 1 h and then next day morning. Results indicated that the overall clinical efficacy of the homeopathic complex (group D) was 94.57% (122/129) with a mean fall of 0.543 ± 0.037°C (0-1.56°C) at 1 h post therapy from its initial temperature. With the continuation of the homeopathic complex there was no increase in rectal temperature. Whereas the clinical efficacy of paracetamol was 86.66% (13/15) with a mean fall of 0.33 ± 0.045°C (0-0.56°C) at 1h post treatment. Nevertheless, rectal temperature returned to normal in both treatment groups (C and D) only when primary cause of fever was attended to.

Clinical Management of Haematuria with Uva ursi

J.P. Varshney (2007 c)

A male Pomeranian dogs aged 10-11 years, with the history of urgency of urination, passing of blood at the end of urination or sometimes reddish urine for 20-25 days showed normal temperature (101.4°F) pollakiuria, dysuria, gross haematuria , tenderness of caudal abdomen , distended urinary bladder on rectal palpation, and normal perineal and bulbospongiosus reflexes. Mean urine residual volume was 16.2 ml kg^{-1}. There was no lesion of canine transmissible veneral tumor. Radiograph and ultrasonogram confirmed distended bladder. Urine analysis revealed turbid, red coloured urine, ammonical smell, alkaline pH (7.8), increased specific gravity (>1.02), presence of erythrocytes (Fig. 12A) ,protein, and struvite crystals (Fig.12B). Cultural examination revealed the preponderance of *E. coli*. The dog was treated with a homeopathic drug *Uva ursi* 3 X) @ 4 drops thrice daily orally for 7 days. With the persistence of microscopic haematuria *Uva ursi* was continued once daily for one week more. Gross haematuria ceased with oral allministration of Uva ursi in 4 days but microscopic haematuria persisted. With continuing therapy for 3 more days, there was significant reduction in microscopic haematuria and pollakiuria also decreased. Complete disappearance of microscopic haematuria took one more week. *Uva ur*si (Bearberry) is an important homeopathic remedy reputed for urinary symptoms particularly frequent urging with blood in urine in humans.

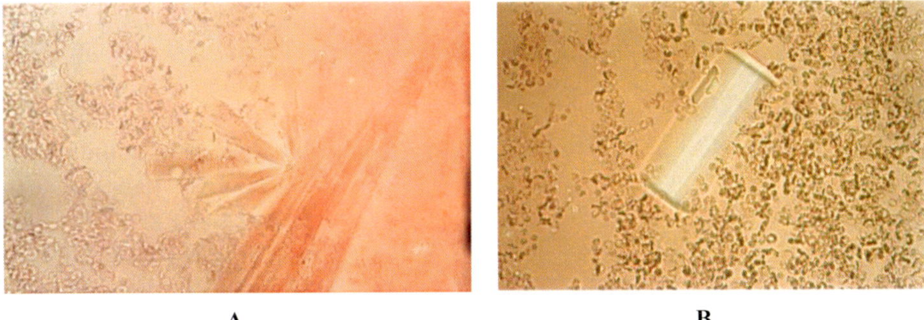

A B

Fig. 12. Urine microscopy of the Pomeranian dog is showing erythrocytes (A) and a crystal of struvite in high power (B).

Clinical Management of Haematuria with a Homeopathic-complex in a Spitz Dog

J.P. Varshney (2007d)

A male Spitz dog, aged 10 years, of a veterinary gyneacologist was referred with the history of passing blood at the end of urination or reddish urine for 5-7 days.Clinical examination at the time of referral revealed normal temperature (101.0 ° F), dysuria, gross haematuria, tenderness over caudal abdomen and arched back. Digital examination was unremarkable. Perineal and bulbospongious reflexes were normal. There was no lesion of canine transmissible veneral tumour on the penis. Radiograph and ultrasonogram showed no evidence of calculi in the kidney, ureters or bladder or enlarged prostates but urinary bladder wall was thickened. Urine analysis revealed turbid red coloured urine, ammonical smell, alkaline pH (8.0), and presence of frank blood . Urine microscopic examination confirmed the abundance of erythrocytes in the urine. Based on history and clinical, urological, radiographic and ultrasonographic examinations, haematuria in this Spitz dog was ascribed to Cystitis. Treatment of the dog was immediately initiated with a homeopathic-complex consisting of *Arsenic alb*., *Crotalus hor*., *China off*., and *Ferrum phos* , *Acid Muriaticum* and *Echinacea agust* each of 200C potency in equal proportions (Healwell E-1 pills- Sintex International Ltd., Kalol, Gujarat,

India). The drug was given @ 4 pills orally four times daily. Gross haematuria began reducing by day 2 post administration of homeopathic –complex and ceased in 4 days but microscopic haematuria persisted even on day 6. With a total of 13 days therapy with the homeopathic –complex haematuria vanished completely. The effect of homeopathic complex in arresting haematuria seems to be due to anti-hemorrhagic properties of *Arsenic alb.*, *Crotalus hor.*, *China off.*, *Ferrum phos* and *Acid Muraaticum* as these drugs have been indicated in cases of various types of bleeding including dark bloody urine in humans.

Clinical Management of haematuric Dog with Cantharis 30c

J.P. Varshney (2013)

A male Labrador dog, aged 8 years, with haematuria, urgency and incontinence of urine for last 10 days was diagnosed with Cystitis. The dog had a history of frequent dribbling of red colored urine and uneasiness for past 10 days. On presentation at the hospital, detailed clinical examination revealed slightly elevated rectal temperature (102.8 ^{0}F), weakness and dullness, frequent urge of urination, pollakiuria, dysuria, stranguria, terminal red colored urine and mild tenderness over caudal abdomen. Rectal examination revealed distended urinary bladder and normal prostate glands. Perineal and bulbo-spongious reflexes were intact. Urine analysis before institution of therapy revealed turbid, foul odor, red color urine with alkaline pH (8.2); proteinuria (++); absence of bile, glucose and ketones; abundance of erythrocytes; 10 pus cell per high power field. Cultural examination showed profuse growth of organisms identified as *E. coli* on the basis of cultural and biochemical characteristics. Plain abdominal and pelvic region X-ray showed distended bladder with no evidence of either renal or urinary bladder calculi or growth. Ultrasonography revealed distended urinary bladder with echogenic moving particles, thickened bladder wall (> 3 mm) and absence of uroliths or tumours(Fig.13).

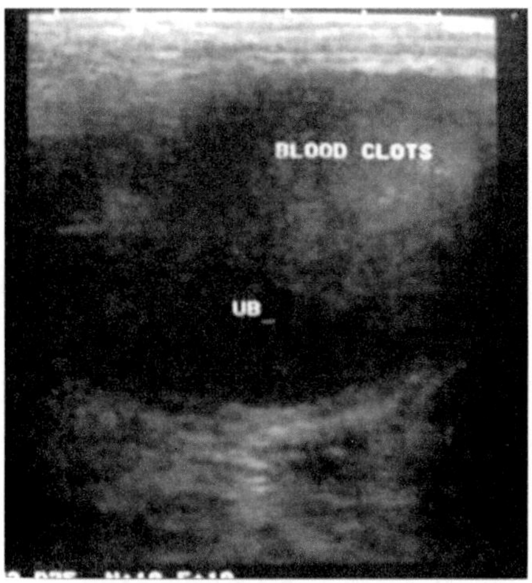

Fig. 13. Ultrasonogram of an eight year old male Labrador with haematuria, urge incontinence showing thickened urinary bladder wall (>3 mm), UB distension and moving echogenic particles.

The basis of diagnosis was clinico-urological examination, preponderance of *E.coli*, RBCs in the urine and ultrasonographic evidence of urinary wall thickness with mixed echo fluid in the urinary bladder. Homeopathic drug Cantharis 30C was chosen on the basis of principal symptoms of urgency, incontinence and haematuria. Therapy with Cantharis 30C, 04 drops in water orally three times a day was instituted. Response was evaluated by clinical examination daily and urinary examination on day 7, 14 and 21 post therapy. The treatment was continued till urine examination showed absence of erythrocytes in the urine. Though gross haematuria ceased on day 7th post therapy, complete recovery with the absence of microscopic haematuria was seen after 21 days of therapy. The dog was subjected to ultrasonographic examination on day 21 when he appeared clinically normal and erythrocytes were absent in the urine.

Clinical management of Cystitis in Dogs with Cantheris

J.P. Varshney (2007 f)

Four dogs with haematuria and incontinence of urine ,refractory to routine treatment ,for last 10-15 days were investigated for disease diagnosis and management. Based on clinico-urological, radiographic and ultrasonographic examinations, the diagnosis was arrived at cystitis. Urine analysis revealed turbid foul odoured reddish urine; varying pH (6 to 8); proteinuria; absence of bile , glucose, ketones; and abundance of RBC (Fig.14) , > 8 WBC/ HPF, 2-4 epithelial cells/HPF and sperms in males. *E.* coli was the predominant microorganism isolated from these cases. Therapy with *Cantheris* 30C @ 2-3 drops` in water orally thrice daily was instituted for a week. Progress was evaluated daily employing clinical examination and assessing the change in the urine. Urological examination was conducted every 3rd day for the presence of erythrocytes and cells. After 3-4 days of cantharis therapy, gross hematuria ceased and symptoms of urge incontinence started regressing. However microscopic hematuria persisted that vanished by day 7 post therapy and symptoms of urge incontinence also ceased. Recovery was uneventful in these dogs treated with *Cantha*ris. Though the therapy was instituted for one week, ultrasonographic evaluation on day 14th post therapy revealed almost normal urinary bladder.` Based on modalities of homeopathic drug that covers symptoms of urge continence, hematuria, dribbling (characteristic of cystitis), *Canthar*is was selected.

Fig. 14. Microscopic examination of the urine of a dog showing preponderance of RBCs revealing hematuria.

Preliminary Observations on Efficacy of Homeopathic Medicines in Field Cases of Bovine Haematuria

Somvanshi (2007)

Haematuric animals were treated with homeopathic medicines, viz *Aconite*, *Bryonia*, *Canthar*is or *Ipecacuanha* 30 c. Eight to ten drops of medicine was given for 10 days orally. Farmers were advised to administer medicine to animals, before offering feed or fodder and to give them rest during the course of treatment. Results indicated that *Ipecacuanha* 30 was most effective (55.55%) followed by *Aconite* 30 (35.71%), *Bryonia* (33.33%) and *Cantheris* (25.00%). Irrespective of medicine, out of 49 cases treated, 20 (40.82%) were cured 15 (30.61%) showed little improvement and 10 (20.41%) failed to show any response. Preliminary efficacy of these medicines was also tested in a limited number of naturally affected haematuric animals procured from Distt. Nainital and maintained under shed conditions at Izatnagar. Physical and microscopic urine examination on 0,5,10, 15 day post treatment was conducted to assess efficacy of different drugs. Results showed that *Ipecacuanha* was most effective (60.00%) followed by *Bryonia* (55.00%), *Cantharis* (40.00%) and *Aconite* (25%). One cow, which was in the advanced state of pregnancy and passing clotted blood, failed to response and succumbed. Another heifer, which was passing dark red urine, revealed drastic transitory improvement. Some animals, which passed straw colored clear urine, were proved microhaematuric. It was also observed that these animals became positive for hematuria after discontinuation of treatment.

Management of Non-specific Diarrhoea Syndrome in Calves with Homeopathic Combination Remedy

Ram Naresh and J.P.Varshney (2004)

Diarrhoea is a common gastrointestinal problem of diversified etiology in calves. The present clinical study was under taken to evaluate homeopathic combination remedy for its anti diarrhoeic efficacy in calves with non-specific diarrhoea. Ten diarrhoeic crossbred calves, aged < 1 month, during rainy season, were treated with a homeopathic combination remedy consisting of *Arsenicum album, Cina, Mercurus corrosivus* and *China off* each 30C potency in equal proportion at the dose rate of 10-15 pills twice daily orally for a period of 7 days.The diarrhoea was characterized by increased frequency (4-6 per day) of soft faeces of white, yellowish or greenish colour with almost normal temperature (99-101°F) and no systemic sign or dehydration. Response to homeopathic therapy was 90% with a mean recovery period of 6.1 days (median 6 days, range 4 to 7 days). Though, clinical improvement became evident from 2nd day onward, drug was continued till complete recovery or a week whichever was earlier.

Clinical Management of Canine Viral Gastroenteritis with a Homeopathic Combination Remedy

J.P. Varshney (2006b)

Viral gastro enteritis caused by canine parvo virus is quite common in dog. The disease in enteric from is characterized by vomiting and watery faces with hematochezia. The present study was conducted to assess the efficacy of a homeopathic combination remedy as a complementary and alternative approach, in the management of canine viral gastroenteritis simulating to Parvo. Forty four pups, aged 2 to 6 months, brought to Referral Veterinary Polyclinic of the Institute with clinical manifestations of vomiting (clear to bile stained), anorexia, loose watery faces mixed with mucus and blood, dehydration, cold extremities, almost normal /slightly subnormal rectal temperature (99.8

to 102^0 F), dullness, weakness and prostration having no detectable cardiac changes were included in the study. Epidemiological considerations, no proper vaccination, clinical manifestations, marked leukopenia due to lymphopenia were suggestive of canine viral gastroenteritis simulating to parvo.

The pups were randomly divided into two groups consisting of 29 pups in group A and 15 pups in group B. Pups of group A were treated with Ringer's lactate (60 ml per kg b.wt., I.V., bid x 3days) and a homeopathic combination remedy (consisting of *Arsenicum album, Podophyllum, Veratrum album, Cina, Mercurius corrosivus,* and *China Off.*) at the dose rate of 4 pills P.O. at 30 min. interval x 2 and then q.i.d for 3 days). While pups of group B were treated with Ringer's lactate (60 ml/per kg b.wt., I.V., bid for 3 days), metoclopramide (0.5-1.0 mg per kg. b.wt., I.M., bid for 3 days) and metronidazole (10.0 mg per kg b.wt., P.O., tid for 3 days). Clinical response and recovery rate (group A- 89.66% and group B-80%) in both the groups was comparable. It appears that homeopathic combination remedy was cost effective as a complementary and alternative approach in the management of viral gastroenteritis.

Management of Gastroenteritis in Pups: A Comparative Clinical Study.

J.P. Varshney (2006c)

Gastroenteritis is a common clinical entity in pups. In poorly managed, unvaccinated pups it is a common clinical manifestation of canine parvo or distemper virus infection. The present study was conducted to assess the efficacy of *Arsenicum album* 30 c as a complementary and alternative medicine in the management of viral gastroenteritis in pups. Twenty pups, aged two to four months, brought to Referral Veterinary Polyclinic of the Institute with clinical manifestations of vomiting just after eating or drinking, anorexia, loose, watery feces mixed with mucus and/or blood, dehydration, cold extremities, almost normal/slightly subnormal rectal temperature (98.8 to 101 ^{0} F), dullness, weakness, prostration, and no detectable cardiac changes, were included in the study Epidemiological considerations - clinical signs of vomiting and loose, watery feces with or without mucus and/or blood ,marked leukopenia due to lymphopenia - were suggestive of canine viral gastroenteritis. The pups were divided into two groups consisting of ten pups in each group. Pups of group A were treated with Ringer's lactate (60 ml per kg body weight, l.V., b.i.d, for 3 days) and *Arsenicum album* 30c at the dose rate of 4 pills PO at thirty minute intervals x 2 and then q.i.d for 3 days). Pups of group B were treated with Ringer's lactate (60 ml/per kg body weight, l.V., b.i.d, for 3 days), ondansetron (0.5-1.0 mg per kg body weight, IV first dose, then PO, b.i.d, for 3 days), a suspension of metronidazole (100 mg per 5 ml) and furazolidone (25 mg per 5 ml) at half to one teaspoonful PO, TID, for 3 days) and cefotaxime

(30 mg/kg body weight IM t.i.d, for 3 days). Clinical response and recovery rate (group A 80.0 %, group B 80.0%) in both the groups was comparable. Total cost of treatment in group A was lower (Rs 35 to 40) than that of group B (Rs.275 to 280). From the preliminary clinical trial it appears that *Arsenicum album* was cost-effective as a complementary and alternative approach in the management of gastroenteritis in pups.

A Preliminary Trial of a Homeopathic Shampoo in the Management of Seborrhoea in Dogs

J.P. Varshney (2007 f)

Eight dogs (German shepherd 4, Dobermann 1, Pomeranian 2, Non descript 1) aged between 1 to 6 years, with the history of excessive scaling and itching referred at Referral Veterinary Polyclinic were selected for the present clinical trial with the full concurrence of the owners. The dogs were regularly dewormed. Clinical examination of the dogs revealed hair matting , excessive diffuse scaling (Fig.15), dryness, rough hairs and itching. The scaling was generalized in most of them. Microscopic examination of skin scrapings was negative for mange mites. Faecal examination was noncommittal.

Seborrheic complex is an important and common dermatological problem of dogs. Based on history, clinical picture and negative skin scrapings, a diagnosis of seborrhoea was arrived at.

The dogs, diagnosed with seborrhoea, were subjected to a homeopathic shampoo consisting of *Sulphur* Q, *Arnica* Q, *Berberis aquifolium* Q and *Calendula* Q, in a base. (Healwell Pet Shampoo – Sintex International Ltd. Kalol). Initially shampoo was applied biweekly for first 2 weeks and then weekly. The dogs were wetted and shampoo was applied, lather was created, left as such for 15-20 min. and then washed and dried. Seborrhoea was characterized by excessive scaling, hair matting, dryness, rough fairs and itching. In first 2 weeks (3-4 applications), scaling reduced and hairs coat was softened. Out of 8 dogs, 6 showed recovery from seborrhea at the end of 4 weeks with the disappearance of scaling and absence of pruritus. In the other 2 dogs scaling disappeared by 7 week. Marked improvement with softening of hairs was noticed with 3-4 applications and Seborrhoea vanished completely in 6 out of 8 dogs in 4 weeks and in remaining 2 dogs in 7 weeks. The homeopathic shampoo was quite effective in the management of seborrhoea and its efficacy could be ascribed to antiseptic activity of *Calendula*; antiscaly, antipruritic and antipsoriosis property of *Berberis aquifoli*um; antiscaling, anti-itching and prophylactic of pus infection property of *Arnica*; and anti-psoric, anti-itching, antiscabies and antiexcoriative activity of *Sulphur* as indicated in humans.

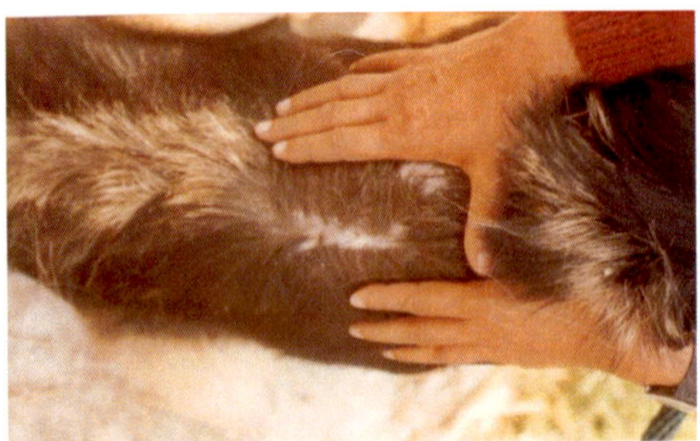

Fig. 15. Excessive diffuse scaling with rough hair coat indicating seborrhoea.

Management of Post partum Anestrus in Dairy Animals with a Homeopathic combination remedy

Harendra Kumar, S.K. Srivastava, M.C. Yadav and J.P. Varshney (2003, 2004)

Parous anestrus crossbred cows (25) and buffaloes (6)were given a homeopathic combination remedy (consisting of *Calcarea phosphorica* , *Aletris farinosa, Aurum Muriaticum natronatum* (*Mur. nat*), *Pulsatilla, Sepia, and Phosphorus* each of 30 C potency in equal proportion) at the dose rate of 15 pills bid orally for 10 days. Animals were observed for onset of behavioral signs of estrus that was confirmed finally on clinico-gynaecological examination. The animals in estrus were inseminated and pregnancy confirmed at 60 days post A.I. Animals, failed to conceive at the induced estrus, were followed for exhibition of signs of estrus. Results revealed that 68% cows and 50% buffaloes exhibited estrus at an average interval of 14.41, and 16.0 days, respectively after treatment. The conception rate in cows was 29.41%, with 1.8 services per conception. The ovarian cyclicity was established in 45 and 33% cattle and buffaloes, respectively.

Management of Infertility in Cows with A Homeo- complex

R. Rajkumar, S.K. Srivastava, M.C. Yadav, V.P. Varshney, J.P. Varshney and H. Kumar (2006)

True anoestrus is the major problem of infertility prevalent in rural cattle population in India.. Many hormonal preparations have been tried on anoestrus animals to induce oestrus and restore the ovarian cyclicity, but the results of hormonal treatments for anoestrus are unsatisfactory. The present investigation was undertaken to evaluate the efficacy of a homeo-complex (comprising of *Calcaria phosphporica* 30C, *Aletris farinosa* 30C, *Pulsatilla* 30C, *Aurum muriatcum natronatum* 30C, *Sepia* 30C and *Phosphorus* 30C in equal proportion) at the dose rate of 15 pills twice daily for 10 days in the management of true anoestrus in crossbred cows. A total of 12 anoestrus cows were randomly divided into two groups comprising of 6 cows in each group. Group I cows were treated orally with homeo- complex and Group II cows were kept as control without any treatment. Results indicated that the treatment was 100% effective in induction of oestrus in anoestrus cows with mean interval of 27.50 ± 5.03 days. All the treated animals conceived and overall conception rate was 54.54% with 1.83 service per conception. In homeopathic complex treated group, increased serum estradiol concentration was observed than the pretreated and control values. The homeo-complex was effective and economical in the treatment of true anoestrus condition in cows.

Clinical Management of Hordeolum / Stye in Dogs with Pulsatilla 200C

J.P. Varshney (2007)

Hordeolum is a non-neoplastic mass involving the eyelids. They are not amenable to medical therapy and require minor surgical intervention. Six cases of chalazion or hordeolum of lower eye lid in dogs were treated with *Pulsatilla* 200c @ 4 pills given orally once in a fortnight. Regression of hordeolum/ chalazion became apparent on day 7 post therapy and it regressed completely by day 14 post therapy in 4 cases (66.66%) with one dose only. Other two cases required repetition of one more dose of *Pulsatilla* 200 c and stye in these cases regressed completely in a total of 21 days without surgical intervention.

Evaluation of Homeopathic Drugs in Clinical Management of Idiopathic Canine Epilepsy

J.P. Varshney (2006 d)

Efficacy of homeopathic drug – *Belladonna*-200c in the clinical management of epilepsy in dogs was evaluated. Ten clinical cases of idiopathic epilepsy in dogs were subjected to homeopathic drugs for the management of epilepsy. Clinical manifestations of epilepsy included behavioural changes during pre-ictal phase; generalized tonic-clonic convulsions, altered muscle tone, paddling, foaming, jaw champing, involuntary urination and defaecation during ictal phase; and dullness in post ictal phase. During the phase of seizure, 3-4 drops of Belladonna 200C were administered orally at 15 min. interval till considerable reduction in seizure activity was evident and then the drug was given orally four times daily. In addition to *Belladonna*, *Cocculus* 6c potency 3-4 drops orally was also used weekly for 3 months in 4 dogs having head shaking syndrome also. In 5 cases, *Belladonna* was continued for 7 months. During seizure phase, reduction in seizure activity with prolongation of inter-ictal phase was observed within an hour in acute crisis. Numbers of fits reduced to 2-3 during first 2 weeks post therapy and then became occasional in next 2 weeks. With continuation of *Belladonna* therapy, no fits were observed during 2-7 months period. However, in 2 cases epileptic fits reappeared within 15-25 days of cessation of therapy. Therefore, Belladonna therapy was started again with which seizure control was again achieved and owners were advised to continue the therapy at least two times daily. Liver specific enzymes (ALT & SAP) monitored at 0 (ALT 25-52 IU/L; SAP 34-62 IU/L), 2 (ALT 30-45 IU/L, SAP 28-70 IU/L) and 4 (ALT 40-68 IU/L, SAP 36-80 IU/L) months post *Belladonna* therapy revealed no significant alterations indicating no induction of liver specific enzymes with homeopathic drugs.

Clinical Management of Babesiosis in dogs with Homeopathic Crotalus horridus 200c

S. Chaudhuri and J.P. Varshney (2007 a)

Homeopathic *crotalus horridus* 200 c was evaluated in 13 clinical cases of babesiosis in dogs, compared with another 20 clinical cases treated with diminazine. The disease is manifested by anorexia, dehydration, temperature, dullness/depression, diarrhea/constipation, pale mucosa, hepatomegaly, vomiting/nausea, splenomegaly, distended abdomen/ascites, yellow colored urine, emaciation/weight loss, and ocular discharge. The diagnosis was based on cytological evidence of *Babesia gibsoni* in freshly prepared blood smears (Fig.16). The dogs were treated with oral Crotalus horridus 200C, 4 pills four times daily for 14 days (n=13) or diminazine aceturate 5 mg /kg single intramuscular injection (n=20). All dogs were administered5% Dextrose saline @ 60 ml/kg intravenously for 4 days. Initial clinical score were similar in both groups and showed similar progressive improvement with the two treatments over 14 days. Parasitaemia also improved in both groups, but hematological values showed no change. No untoward reactions were observed. It appears that *Crotalus horridus* is as effective in causing clinical recovery in moderate cases of canine babesiosis caused by *Babesia gibsoni* as the standard drug diminazine. Large scale randomized trials are indicated for more conclusive results. In homeopathy , *Crotalus horridus*, *Phosphorus, Ficus religiosa*, *China officinalis* and *Milleforlium* have been recommended in the treatment of babesiosis in cattle. *Crotalus horridus* is a drug of choice for hemorrhagic diathesis. The properties of *C. horridus* matched well with the clinical manifestations of babesiosis in dogs.

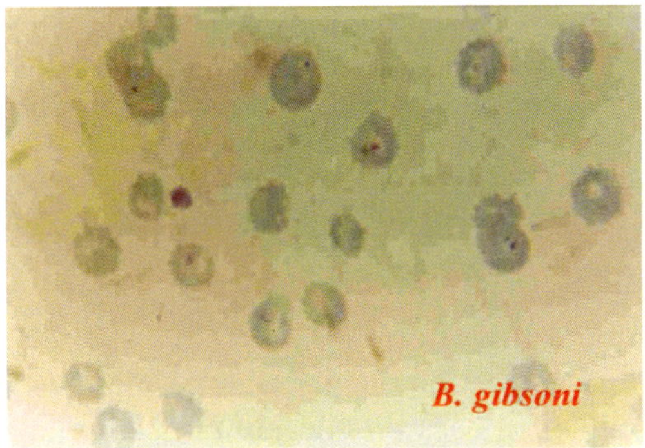

Fig. 16. Blood smear cytology of a dog suffering from babesiosis is revealing Babesia gibsoni infection

Clinical management of anaemia associated with babesiosis in dogs with Trinitrotoluenum 200 C

S. Chaudhuri and J.P. Varshney (2007 b)

Anaemia is an important accompaniment of canine babesiossis, caused by *Babesia gibsoni*, owing to hemolysis. Anaemia is manifested as marked weakness, yellowish colored urine, weight loss, exertion, dullness, depression, pale mucosa, panting on slight exertion, loss of appetite, dehydration besides other symptoms associated with babesiosis (fever, hepatomegaly, splenomegaly, nausea/vomiting, diarrhea. Constipation or ocular discharge).The study was conducted on 18 dogs in varying age groups (4 months to 60 months) confirmed with anemia (based on hemogram) and cytological evidence of *B. gibsoni* infection. The dogs were grouped in two groups A (consisting of 12 babesiosis affected dogs) and group B (considting of 6 babesiosis affected dogs).Initial hemogram was characterized by low hemoglobin (A 5.42±).54 g/dl, range 3.0-8.0g; B7.37±0.55 g/dl,range 6.0- 9.0 g/dl),packed cell volume(A 16.90±1.56%, range9.0-24.0%, B 22.0±1.61%, range 18.0-28.0%), and total erythrocyte count (A 2.63±0.26 million/mm^3, range1.69- 4.86 million/mm^3 , range, B 3.29±0.33 million/mm^3, range 2.51 - 4.62 million/mm^3). Dogs of group A were treated with *Trinitrotoluenum* 200c @ 4 pills orally four times a day for 14 days alongwith single intramuscular injection of diminazine aceturate @ 5.0 mg/kg body wt. and dogs of group B were treated with diminazene aceturate @ 5.0 mg/kg body wt. once intramuscularly only. Dogs of both groups were evaluated for their hemogram at day 0,3,7 and 14 post therapy. The results indicated that the dogs of group A and B differed significantly ($p<0.05$) on day 14th with respect to hemoglobin, packed cell volume and total erythrocyte count indicating that that homeopathic *Trinitrotoluenum* assisted in improving the erythrocyte in dices in cases of canine babesiosis , caused by *B. gibsoni*. TNT was a chosen because of destruction of erythrocytes leading to anemia is the main symptom of TNT in healthy subjects and it is also a main problem in babesiosis having similarity.

Clinical Management of Squamous Metaplasia with Thuja in a Dog

J.P. Varshney and O.P. Paliwal (2007)

A male non-descript dog (eight month old) with normal temperature (101°F), normal pulse (88 per minute) and normal respiration (20 per minute), alertness, normal appetite, but small whitish nodular masses on buccal mucosa, mouth commissures and lips (Fig.17), ptyalism, no oral bleeding was presented for treatment. Haemogram was almost normal (Hb 9.8 g/dl, TLC 8350 per mm3, Neutrophils 50%, lymphocyte 32%, monocyte 2%) except eosinophil counts (16%). Histopathological examination of the biopsied tissue revealed keratinization of epidermis. The underlying epithelium exhibited hyperplastic changes of squamous appearance and at places squamous metaplasia leading to a diagnosis of squamous metaplasia. The dog was given homeopathic drug *Thuja* 200 @ 5-6 pills orally thrice daily. With three weeks therapy with *Thuja* 200 overgrowths regressed completely.

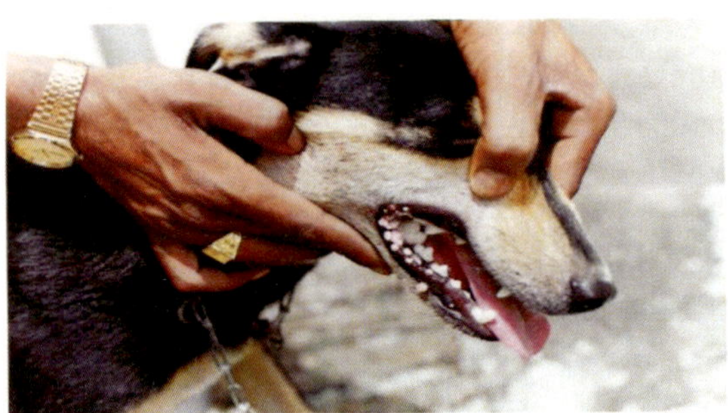

Fig.17. Whitish nodular masses on buccal mucosa, mouth commissures and lips in a nondescript dog diagnosed with squamous metaplasia.

Therapeutic Management of Cutaneous Warts in A Heifer By Thuja

R. Somvanshi and R.D. Sharma (2007)

A non-descript heifer, affected with horny nodular, tumour like growth in the front of lower jaw was treated with homeopathic Thuja 30 (10 drops orally for a period of 10 days). On microscopic examination, finger-like projections were diagnosed as fibropapilloma with a tendency of regression. Soon, tumour growth disappeared and the animal was recovered completely.

Evaluation of Anti-Haemorrhagic Efficacy of a Homeo-complex in the Management of Haemorrhagic Crisis Associated with Canine Ehrlichiosis

Ajay Kumar and J.P. Varshney (2005)

Haemorrhagic syndrome in chronic severe ehrlichiosis in some breeds of dog is a serious clinical problem warranting emergency management failing which, survivability of the dog is threatened. Haemostats currently in use are of little value in these cases owing to severe thrombocytopenia. In homeopathy, drugs such as *Arsenic album, Crotalus hor., China off, Ferum phos and Acid muriaticum* have been claimed to have good anti-haemorrhagic efficacy. Nevertheless, these drugs have not been evaluated in dogs with haemorrhagic syndrome associated with ehrlichiosis. Therefore, the present study was undertaken to evaluate the efficacy of a homeo-complex in the management of haemorrhagic crisis associated with canine monocytic ehrlichiosis. A total of 33 dogs with canine monocytic ehrlichiosis showing epistaxis (Fig 18A) , gastrointestinal hemorrhages (Fig.18C) or skin petechiae (Fig.18B), were used in this trial. The dogs were randomly divided into four groups. They were treated with Doxycycline alone, doxycycline with prednisolone, doxycycline with a homeocomplex (consisting of *Arsenic alb. Crotalus hor, China off, Ferrum phos, Ehinacea agust, Acid muriaticum* each of 200C potency in equal proportions), and doxycycline with haemocoagulase in group A, B, C, and D respectively.

The earliest arrest of haemorrhages was observed in group A (Doxycycline alone) on day 4 (40% cases); group B (Doxycycline with Prednisolone) on day 2 (22.22% cases); group C (Doxycycline with Homeo-complex) on day 1 (20% cases); and group D (Doxycycline with Haemocoagulase) on day 4 (50% cases) with an overall efficacy of 60%, 88.88%, 90% and 75% respectively on day 5 post therapy indicated the superiority of the homeo-complex . An increase of 63.14% in platelet count in this group on day 7 post treatments further substantiated the superiority of the homeo-complex.

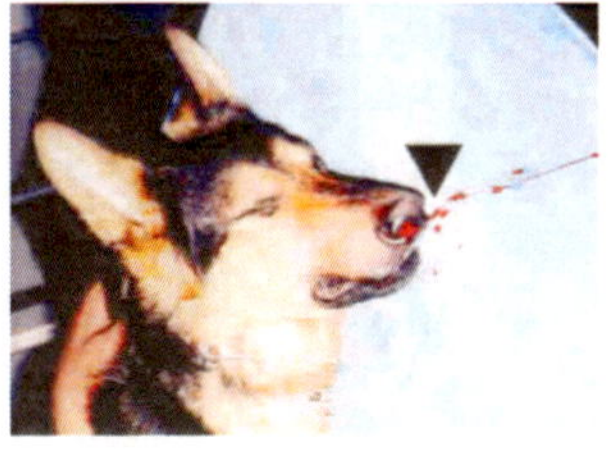

A

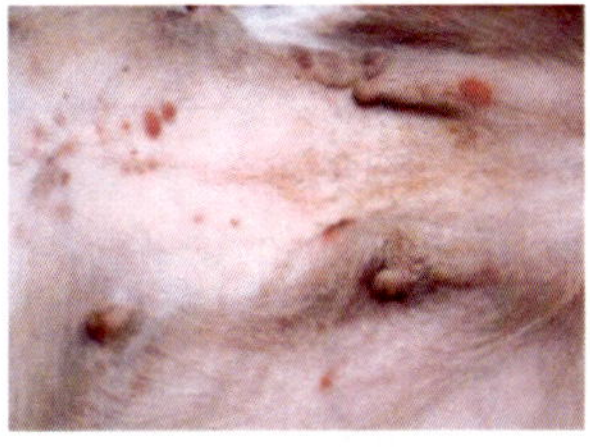

B

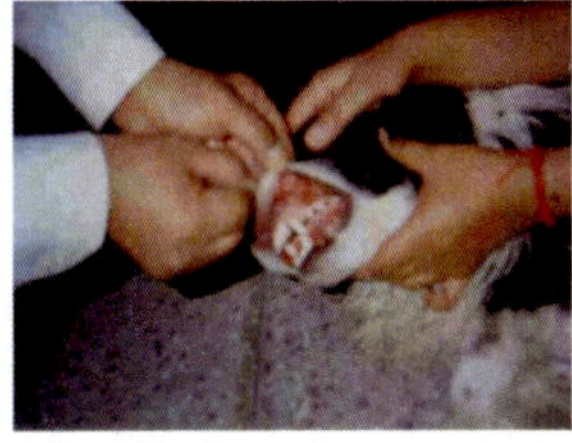

C

Fig.18. Dogs suffering from Ehrlichiosis showing epistaxis (A), skin petechae (B) and haemorrhages on gums (C).

Clinical Management of Tachycardia in Dogs with Abies nigra

Bendangla Changkija and J.P. Varshney (2005)

Three cases of narrow 'QRS' tachyarrhythmia in dogs (Pomeranian 2, non descript 1), aged 8 to 30 months, confirmed with repeated electro-cardiograms (increased heart rate 280 to 360 bpm ; highly variable 'R-R' interval 0.10 to 0.32 sec; shorter 'P-R' interval 0.02 to 0.04 sec, and short QRS duration 0.02 to 0.03 sec) were treated with homeopathic drug - *Abies nigra* 30C @ 4 drops orally q.i.d. for 3-7 days . It is quite evident from the ECG that heart rate decreased from 360 to 210 (Case No.1), 280 to 240 (Case NO.2) and from 300 to 280 (case No3) bpm, with an increase in 'QRS' (case no.1 from 0.02 to 0.04 s, case no.2 from 0.03 to 0.04 s, case no.3 from 0.03 to 0.04 s),P-R interval (Case no.1 from 0.02 to 0.04 s, case no.2 from 0.04 to 0.08 s, case no. 2 from 0.04 to 0.08 s), ST interval (case no. 1 from 02 to 04 s, case no.2 from 0.02 to 0.02 s, case no. 3 from 0.02 to 0.06 s) and QT interval (case no. 1 from 0.10 to 0.12, case no.2 from 0.12 to 0.12 s, case no.3 from 0.12 to 0.16 s) 15 minutes post therapy. The continuation of therapy further improved the cardiac function..

Clinical Management of Bradycardia in a Non-Descript Dog with Abies nigra.

Bendangla Changkija and J.P. Varshney (2007)

Though bradycardia often constitutes a normal finding in atheletic dogs, it has been associated with administration of various drugs, trauma, diseases of CNS, organic diseases of sinus node, hypothermia, hyperkalemia, hypothyroidism, toxaemia and diseases that increases vagal tone . Asymptomatic bradycardia or bradyarrhythmias are benign and insignificant but symptomatic bradycardia assumes greater significance for its impending threat of heart failure or death. A male non descript dog , four and half year old,with marked weakness and short breath was found having severe bradycardia (slow heart rate 40 bpm , slightly variable 'R-R' interval 1.04 – 1.44 second and almost constant 'P-R' interval 0.06 – 0.08 second). Pending final diagnosis, the dog was immediately treated with *Abies nigra* 30c @ four drops orally q.i.d. for seven days and fluid support (5% DNS @ 60 ml/kg b.wt. I.V.). Electrocardiogram was taken initially, 15 minutes post therapy and on day 4 to measure the impact of *Abies nigra* on wave forms and durations. The results indicated that one dose of *Abies nigra* increased heart rate from 40 to 60 bpm. With the continuation of therapy heart rate further improved to 80 bpm.

Effect of Calendula officinalis in Burn Wounds of Calves and Heifers

Aswathy Gopinathan, A.M. Pawde and Kiranjeet Singh (2007)

Debudding wounds in calves and branding wounds in heifers were selected as model for burn wounds in this study. Four groups comprising a minimum of six animals each were treated with the following medicaments such as Calendula glycerine (CG) alone (group I), CG+Himax (CG+H group II), CG+calendula ointment (CG + CO group III) and CG+Lorexane (CG + L group IV). Clinical and haematobiochemical studies were conducted at day zero and subjective wound evaluation was conducted subsequently at weekly intervals. Area of wound contraction was measured at weekly intervals. CG alone was commendable in healing burn wounds followed by its combination with Lorexane. Combination of CG with Himax or CO showed less wound contraction but the wounds remained dry at the end of observation period. The paraffin base of Calendula ointment and that of Himax impaired healthy healing.

Therapeutic evaluation of homeopathic treatment for canine oral papillomatosis

P.A.A. Raj , S. Pavulraj, M.A. Kumar, S. Sangeetha, R. Shamugapriya and S. Sabithabanu (2020)

A placebo controlled study was conducted to evaluate the ameliorative potential of homeopathic drugs in combination (*Sulfur* 30c, *Thuja* 30c, *Graphites* 30c, and *Psorinum* 30c) in 16 dogs affected with oral papillomatosis. Homeopathic combination remedy and placebo drug (distilled water) was administered orally twice daily for 15 days. The homeopathic treatment group showed early recovery with a significant reduction in oral lesions reflected by clinical score ($p<0.001$) in comparison to placebo-treated group. Oral papillomatous lesions regressed in the homeopathic group between 7 and 15 days, whereas regression of papilloma in the placebo group occurred between 90 and 150 days. The homeopathic treated group was observed for 12 months post-treatment period and no recurrence of oral papilloma was observed.

Homeopathic Treatment of Trauma, Abscess and Papillomatosis in Trachemys dorbigni

B.Scardoeli, F.B. Narita,S.R. Pinheiro, A von. Ancken and C.de P. Cidéli de Paula Coelho (2021)

Mechanical trauma, bacterial and viral infections are common in *Trachemys dorbigni* when in captivity. One month old *Trachemys dorbigni* (weight 6 g) with lethargy, hyporexia, locomotor difficulty due to edema and necrotic process in the right anterior limb, was treated with 2 globules of *Arnica montana* 6CH, diluted in the contact water, every 8 hours, for 7 days and 2 globules of *Avena sativa* 6CH, every 12 hours, for 5 days. After 7 days, the patient was active, normoretic, with weight gain and decreased edema and necrosis of the right anterior limb but showed a rigid abscess in the right cervical region. Treatment with a single dose of 2 globules of *Silicea* 6CH and 2 globules of *Arnica montana* 6CH, diluted in the contact water, every 24 hours, showed complete regression in 4 days. After 11 days the animal showed papilloma and plastron infection and was treated with the administration of 2 globules of *Thuja occidentalis* 12CH, diluted in the contact water, every 24 hours for 3 days, with total remission of the lesions.

The Effect of the Pulsatilla 30C as Homeopathy for Ophthalmic Diseases with Concomitant Separation Anxiety

H.K.Hwang, H.G. Yang, M.S. Kim andN.S.Kim (2011)

Homeopathic *Pulsatilla* 30c was evaluated in 4 clinical cases of ophthalmic complications with concomitant separation anxiety in dogs.. Among the material medical remedy of homeopathy, the *Pulsatilla* is used as homeopathic remedy for ocular problems, earache, cough, cold, and anxiety from lost attention. These dogs were completely cured of physical and behavior problem within 10 days. On following up, any clinical signs were not observed at one month after the last therapy.

Treatment of canine atopic dermatitis with a commercial homeopathic remedy: A single-blinded, placebo-controlled study

D. W. Scott, W. H. Miller Jr. D. A. Senter, C. P. Cook, J. E. Kirker, and S. M. Cobb (2002)

A commercial homeopathic remedy and a placebo were administered orally as individual agents to 18 dogs with atopic dermatitis. The pruritus was reduced by less than 50% in only 2/18 dogs; 1 of these dogs was receiving the homeopathic remedy, the other was receiving the placebo. One dog vomited after administration of the homeopathic remedy. All dogs had nonseasonal pruritus of 1 y to 7.5 y duration. They were free of bacterial and yeast infections and ectoparasites, based on physical examination, negative skin scrapings, and negative cytological examination. All dogs had moderate to severe pruritus. The pruritus of all dogs was known to respond completely to anti-inflammatory doses of glucocorticoids. The dogs had been treated previously with 1 to 8 nonsteroidal antipruritic agents (including antihistamines, omega-3/ omega-6 fatty acids, misoprostol, and pentoxifylline) and had failed to respond. The dogs were treated with the commercial homeopathic remedy (Skin and

Seborrhea Remedy; HomeoPet, West Hampton Beach, New York) during the first 3 week of the trial, followed by a placebo (the ethanol-containing vehicle in which the active ingredients are suspended) for the second 3 wk. The dose of both products was 10 drops/dog, q8h, by mouth. The homeopathic remedy contained *sulfur, staphysagria, psorinum, graphites, and arsenicum album*. Only one dog (case 2) had a repeated and sustained "fair" response to the commercial homeopathic remedy. Another dog (case 6) had a repeated and sustained "fair" response to the placebo. When the ethanol was removed from the placebo, the beneficial effect was lost. Four dogs (cases 4, 9, 10, and 17) were thought to have a "fair" or "good" response to the commercial homeopathic remedy during the initial 3-week treatment period, but they did not have a repeatable response during the 30-day period. All other dogs received no benefit from either product. In conclusion, under the conditions of our study, the commercial homeopathic remedy was not effective for the treatment of CAD.

Clinical Management of Vesicular and Pustular Dermatitis in Goats with Homeopathic Drugs

B.K. Choudhury, S. Choudhury, J. Meher, M. Dash, S. Bagh, B.K. Behera and S. Ratha (2024)

The present clinical study was conducted on 40 goats suffering from pustular dermatitis simulating to goat pox in Kantamal Block of Boudh district in Odisha state. The illness of the goats was clinically characterized by fever (mean temperature 104.5^{0}F), lethargy, ophthalmic and nasal discharge, anorexia, small red spots(roseola), papules, nodules, vesicles (predominantly seen on muzzle, eyelids, ears, mouth and udder), and pustules in many cases. Based on epidemiological considerations (contagiousness and quick spread) and clinical symptoms, the disease in goats was diagnosed as vesicular and pustular dermatitis simulating to goat pox. The affected goats were randomly divided into two groups (A and B) consisting of 20 goats in each group. Goats of group- A were simply isolated and kept in secluded place with all hygienic measure and served as control. While goats of group-B were treated with homeopathic *Variolinum* 200 C and *Kali muraticum* 200 C @ five drops each given orally thrice daily for predetermined period of five days. The response was evaluated in both the groups on day 7th. Fever persisted; nodular, vesicular and pustular lesions became suppurative in many goats with death of 5 goats in group -A. While appetite returned with a decrease in nasal and ocular discharge and various degree of healing of vesicular and pustular lesions in 16 goats of group-B (given homeopathic drugs) making the recovery rate as 80%. Though further studies are needed, the use of *Variolinum* 200C and *Kali muraticum* 200C in cases of vesicular and pustular dermatitis in goats seems encouraging.

Therapeutic efficacy of homeopathy (Crotalus horridus) and allopathy (Doxycycline) drugs in Canine Ehrlichiosis

G. D. Risheen, K. K Walwadker, K.K. Mishra and S. Shrivastava (2022)

Canine ehrlichiosis is an earmarked rickettesial disease caused by an intracytoplasmic parasite *Ehrlichia canis*, seen in circulating monocytes and lymphocytes. It is characterized by fever, neurological, ocular signs and bleeding through natural orifices in the form of epistaxis, hematemesis and dermal petechiae, lymphadenomegaly, splenomegaly. The present therapeutic trial included four groups, Healthy group as control (Group I), Allopathy (Doxycycline) (Group II), Homeopathy (Crotalus horridus-200C) (Group III) and Allopathy +Homeopathy group (Group IV). The resolution of symptoms in dogs along with time duration for hemato-biochemical parameters to return to normal values, were used as criteria for deciding therapeutic efficacy of different drugs. Present study revealed that combination therapy, group III (Allopathy +Homeopathy) is better as compared to group I (Allopathy) or group II (Homeopathy) as the values of haemogram and thrombocyte count increased and the monocyte count, liver and values returned to normal at a faster rate in comparison to other groups.

Case Study: Canine Bladder Tumour (Transitional Cell Carcinoma)

J.P. Varshney and S. Swaminarayan (2018)

An adult (3.5 years old) Labrador bitch (Fig.18) was presented at the hospital with the history of blood in urine for about 80 days. Clinical examination of the dog revealed fever (10.40F) , vomiting. difficulty in passing urine, red colored urine , straining to defecate with soft stools, a small palpable raised area of urinary bladder on digital rectal examation. Ultrasound examination confirmed a small irregular area of mucosa adjacent to the neck of bladder (trigone area), hyperechoic shreads in mucosal margins with anechoic fluid in urinary bladder. Urine examination showed preponderance of erythrocytes, transitional cells and organisms leading to the diagnosis of tumor of urinary bladder (most probably Transitional Cell Carcinoma) and with the consent of the owner the dog was treated with Calcarea carbonica 30C once fortnightly. Symptoms started resolving within 10 days of the treatment. Therapy continued and a little difficulty in urination with a few drops of blood was reported again after 59 days.

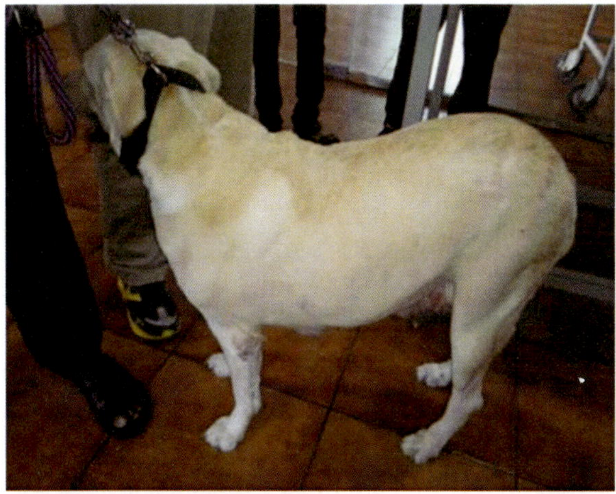

Fig. 19. An adult Labrador bitch with urinary bladder tumour (akin to transitional cell carcinoma) responded to *Calcarea carbonica* 30 c.

Management of Transitional Cell Carcinoma in dogs with Homeopathic Calcarea carbonica

J.P. Varshney (2024 a)

Five client owned adult dogs with the history of persistent dribbling of blood/ red colored urine for 3 to 13 week, refractory to allopathic treatment ,were presented at the hospital for diagnosis and treatment during last eight years. Detailed clinical examination revealed normal vitals, alertness, dribbling of blood from the penis/vagina with or without urination. Haemogram was within normal range except marginal leucocytosis in one case. Blood biochemistry panel (BUN, serum creatinine, random blood glucose, ALT) was within normal range. Survey radiography ruled out uroliths. Abdominal sonography showed variable size of irregular area of mucosa adjacent to the neck of bladder (trigone area), hyperechoic shreds in mucosal margins , anechoic fluid in urinary bladder and thickened wall of urinary bladder (Fig.20 and 21). Urine examination revealed a lot of erythrocytes, large number of pleomorphic epithelial cells having high nuclear to cytoplasmic ratio akin to transitional cell carcinoma (Fig.24) . Urine culture revealed the growth of *E. coli*. Based on history clinical picture, ultrasound examination, and urinary examination, the cases were tentatively diagnosed with transitional cell carcinoma with cystitis. With the consent of owners the treatment was started with *Calcarea carbonica* 30C fortnightly for two occasions followed by *Calcarea carbonica* 200 C monthly for 8 months with monthly clinical evaluation. Because of associated *E.coli* infection the dogs were also given *Cantharis* 30 C (4 pills three times daily for 15 days) .At the end of 8th month treatment the dogs were again evaluated clinically, ultrasonographically (Fig.22) and pneumocystographically (Fig.23) for the changes in tumor size and urologically for the presence or absence of erythrocytes and transitional cells. Post therapy evaluation revealed dark but not red colored urine (microscopic hematuria with 150-200 RBCs per high power field), regression of clinical signs at the end of 2nd week; 4-6 RBCs per high power field and absence of *E. coli* in the urine at the end of 4th week; and complete regression of tumor mass with normal clinical and urological findings at the end of 8th month. This report provides sonographic and pneumocystographic evidences of the efficacy of *Calcarea carbonica* in the management of urinary bladder tumor akin to transitional cell carcinoma in dogs.

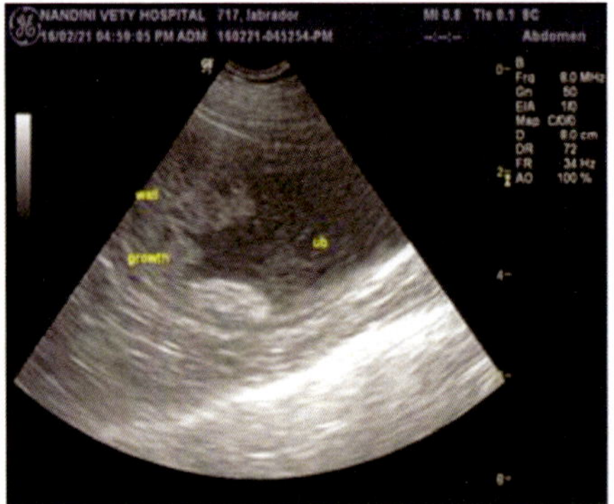

Fig. 20. Ultrasonogram of a six year old Labrador bitch with haematuria showing irregular broad based echogenic mass attached to bladder wall and projecting in to lumen of urinary bladder in trigone area suggesting tumor possibly transitional cell carcinoma.

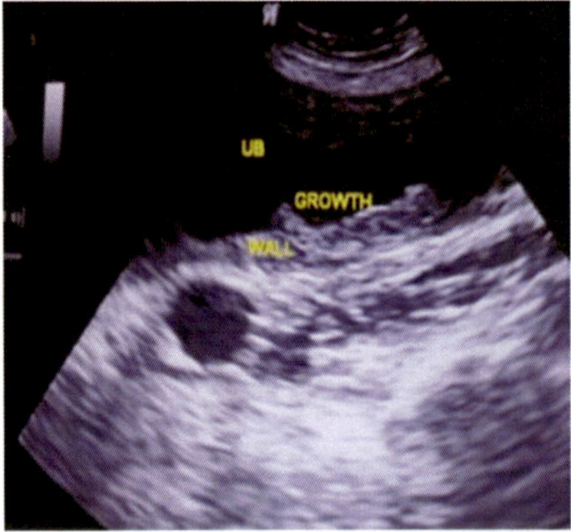

Fig. 21. Ultrasonogram of a 10 year old male Dachshund with dribbling of blood at the time of referral showing irregular broad based echogenic mass attached to bladder wall and projecting in to lumen of urinary bladder in trigone area suggesting tumor possibly transitional cell carcinoma.

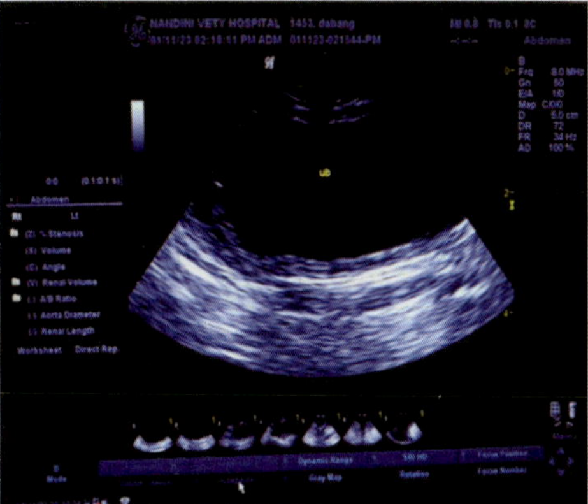

Fig. 22. 2nd Ultrasonogram of the male Dachshund after eight months of therapy with *Calcarea carbonica* showing a clear urinary bladder with no echonegic mass attached to its wall.

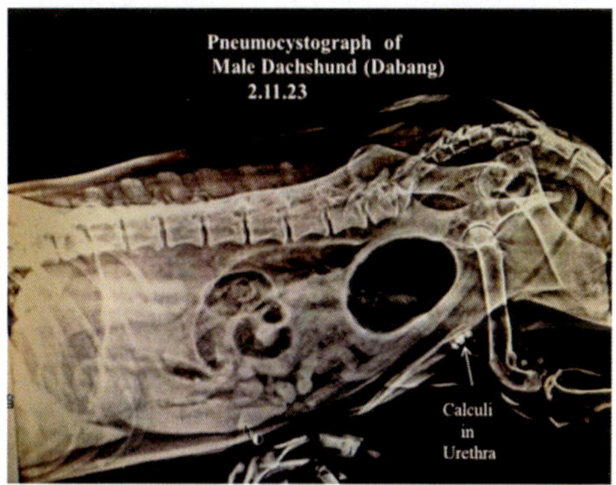

Fig. 23. Penumocystograph of the male Dachshund after eight months of therapy with ***Calcarea carbonica*** showing clear air filled urinary bladder, smooth bladder wall with no mass attached to it. Three small calculi are visible in penile urethra.

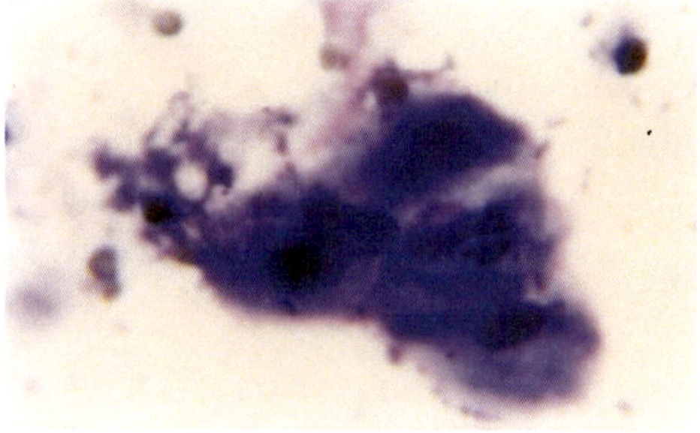

Fig. 24. Transitional cells in the urine of a dog.

Clinical Management of Osteo-arthritis in dogs with a Homeopathic Combination Remedy

J.P. Varshney (2016)

Twenty client owned dogs with hind limb lameness, inability to get up unassisted, reluctance to move, and/or altered behavior for last one to five month were diagnosed with osteo-arthritis of Hip and/or Stiffle joint (s) on radiological evaluation (Fig.25A) and were treated with a homeopathic combination remedy consisting of *Arnica M.*30C, *Ruta G.*,30C, *Rhus Tox* 30C, *Hypericum P.* 30C, *Kali Phos* 30C and *Mag Phos* 30C in equal proportions at the dose rate of 4 pills four times daily orally for 4 weeks. Clinical response was monitored weekly and radiological evaluation was done at the end of 4th week .There was progressive decline in clinical score from 1st to 4th week and radiographic recovery (Fig.25B) was marked at the end of 4th week with an improvement in quality of life. Two of the 20 dogs were dropped from the study as they collapsed on day 4th and 5th post therapy due to hyperthermia (heat stroke).Mean clinical score declined progressively from 14.4 ± 0.53 (range 11.0 to 18.0, median 13.5) on day 0 to 12.55 ±0.41(range 10.0 to 17.0, median 12.0) at the end of 1st week to 10.05 ±0.44 (range 7.0 to 14.0, median 10.0) at the end of 2nd week to 6.5 ±0.23 (range 5.0 to 8.0, median7.0) at the end of 3rd week to 4.72 ± 0.135 (range 4.0 to 6.0, median 5.0) at the end of 4th week) and reached almost at normal level. Improvement in clinical score was associated with radiological evidence of reduction in degenerative joint fill up and increase in joint space at the end of four week therapy (Fig.25B). Scoring of clinical outcome at the end of 4th week therapy (table1) indicated that dogs having clinical signs for shorter period at the time of referral had better clinical outcome as compared to those having clinical signs for longer period. The effectiveness of the homeopathic complex in the management of osteoarthritis of hips/stifles/both in dogs could be ascribed to *Arnica* for its effect on traumatic injuries; *Ruta* for its action on periosteum and cartilage where there is tendency of deposit formation in joints; *Hypericum* for excessive pain in hind limbs; *Rhus tox* for its action on joints; *Kali phos* for lameness in extremities which aggravates on exertion- a common accompaniment in osteo-arthritis in dogs ; and *Mag Phos* for its ability to increase bone density or arrests bone loss .

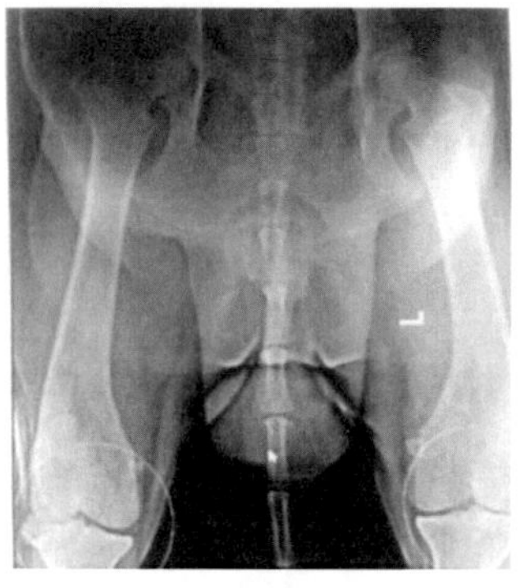

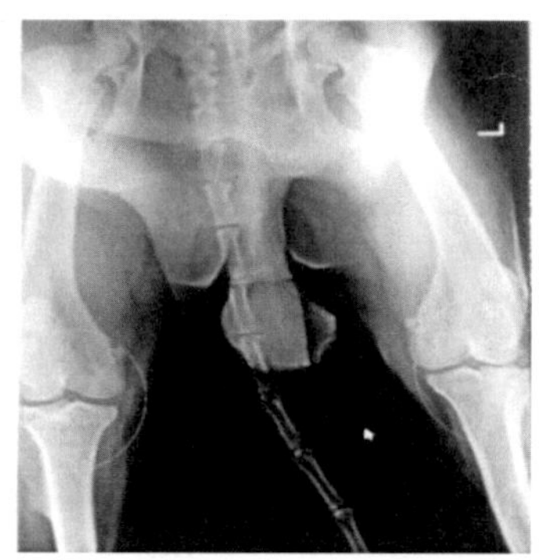

A B

Fig. 25. Radiograph of an adult German Shepherd at A showing osteoarthritis of both stifle joints.Joint space is markedly narrowed in both stifle joints (A- marked with white circle). Radiograph of the same German Sepherd at B after four weeks of homeopathic therapy is showing marked improvement in joint space of both stifle joints (B- marked with white circle).

Table 1: Duration of lameness before therapy and subjective scoring of clinical outcome one month post Homeopathic therapy

Sl.No.	Duration of lameness at the time of referral (Months)	Number of Observations	Subjective grading of clinical outcome Post therapy Mean±S.E
1.	0-1 month	03	3.0± 0
2.	1-2 month	04	2.75±0.25
3	2-3 month	05	2.25±0.20
4	3-4 month	03	2.0± 0.0
5	4-5 month	03	1.66±0.33

0= worse / no change, 1= improvement, 2= great improvement, 3= returned to normal /near to normal

Clinical Management of Suppurative-arthritis in a crossbred calf with a Homeopathic Combination Remedy after drainage

J.P. Varshney (2024 b)

A crossbred orphan calf (one month old) was referred at the hospital with the history of right fore limb lameness for last 10 days. Clinical examination at the time of referral revealed marked lameness of right fore limb ; hot , painful and soft swelling on right carpal joint (Fig.26 A) : anorexia; and increased temperature (103.4 ^{0} F). Aseptic aspiration of the right carpal joint yielded approximately 30 ml pus (Fig. 26B) . Leukocytosis with neutrophilia (TLC 18,000 /mm3, with 65% neutrophils) was evident on blood examination. The calf was diagnosed with suppurative arthritis and treated with a homeopathic combination remedy consisting of *Arnica M.*30c, *Ruta G.*,30c, *Rhus Tox* 30c,

Hypericum P. 30c, *Kali Phos* 30c and *Mag Phos* 30c(all in equal proportions) at the dose rate of 10 pills four times daily orally for seven days. Because of suppuration the calf was also given *Hepar sulph* 30 c (10 pills three times daily for first seven days. Post therapeutic evaluation on 7th day revealed marked reduction in swelling, lameness and pain with resumption of feed intake. The therapy continued for one more week. Second evaluation revealed further improvement (Fig.26C) but still occasional limping. The therapy was continued further for two more weeks. Evaluation at the end of 4th week therapy was much encouraging with almost no lameness, normal vitals, good appetite but the carpal joint was a little bit bigger than the left carpal joint. There was progressive decline in clinical score from 1st to 4th week with an improvement in quality of life.

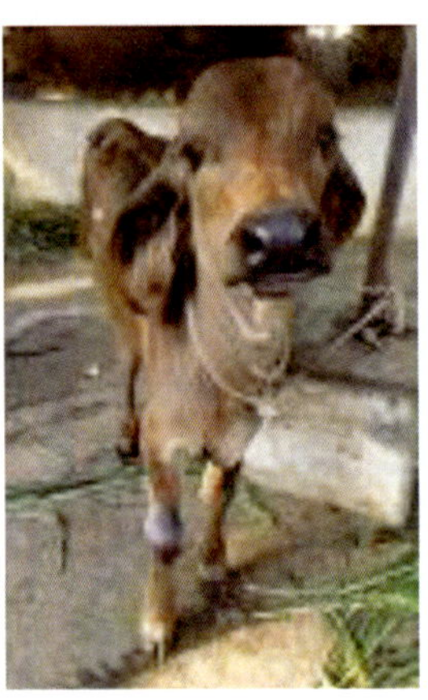

A

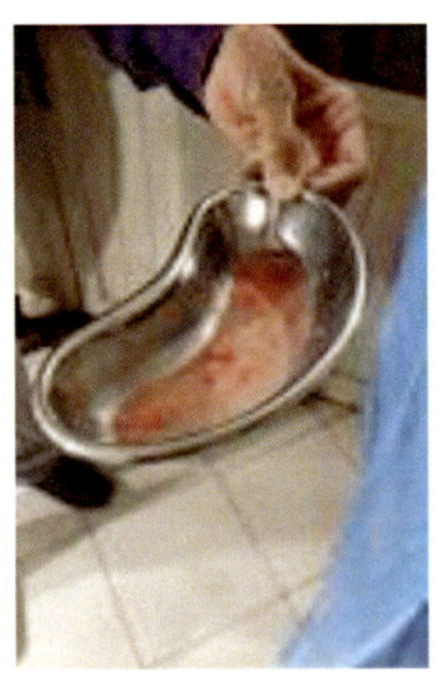

B

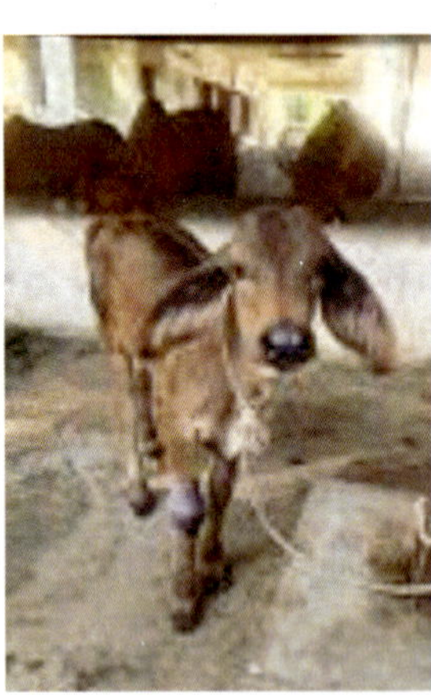

C

Fig. 26. Showing suppurative arthritis in an orphan crossbred calf. A. Swollen right carpal joint. B. Aseptic Needle aspiration yielded pus making the diagnosis of suppurative arthritis. C. Calf showing reduction in swelling and improvement with homeopathic treatment.

Clinical Management of aural hematoma with Arnica montana and Hamamelis virginica

J.P. Varshney (2024 c)

Aural hematoma is described as surgical condition manageable by surgical intervention with a fair chance of recurrence. Twenty four cases of aural hematoma (Cocker Spaniels 4, Beagles 5, German shepherd 3, Labrador 3, Pomeranian 4, spitz 1, cat 02 and rabbit 02) were subjective to homeopathic treatment (group A) with the consent of the owners. Of these, three cases in dogs were of recurrence after surgical intervention. .Another four cases of aural hematoma (Cocker Spaniel 1, German Shepherd 2, Beagle 1) remained without any treatment for two month because of owners indecisiveness and served as control (group B). All 24 cases were clinically characterized by blood-filled subcutaneous hot to touch fluctuant swelling on the pinna (Fig 27 A, 28 A), separation of the auricular cartilage and skin ,drooping ear (Fig.28 C), head shaking and ear scratching . Needle aspiration in all cases revealed a sero-hemorrhagic, fibrotic rich fluid confirming hematoma . Aural hematomas are ascribed to traumatic rupture of blood capillaries. Animals of group A were treated with homeopathic *Arnica montana* 30 c(2 to 4 drops PO BID) and *Hamamelis virginiana* 30 c (2-4 drops PO BID) daily till recovery with weekly clinical evaluation. Reduction in the size of lesion started in 7 to 21 days (Fig.27 B, 28 B). Complete resolution of the hematoma took place in variable period of time ranging from 21 to 63 days depending on the size of the lesion. In two cases (One Labrador and one German Shepherd) fibrosis occurred leading to malformation of the pinna. Whereas , the size of aural hematoma did not regressed but increased in dogs of group B.

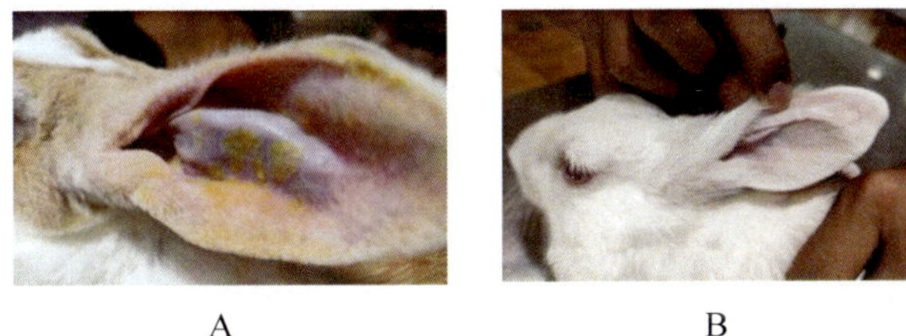

A B

Fig. 27. Photographs of the rabbit affected with aural hematoma and its recovery on *Arnica* and *Hamamelis*. A. Left ear pinna hematoma on day 0 (day of referral). B. Left ear pinna of the same rabbit (at A) on day 14 post therapy with homeopathic *Arnica* and *Hamamelis* showing complete resolution of hematoma with out any fibrosis.

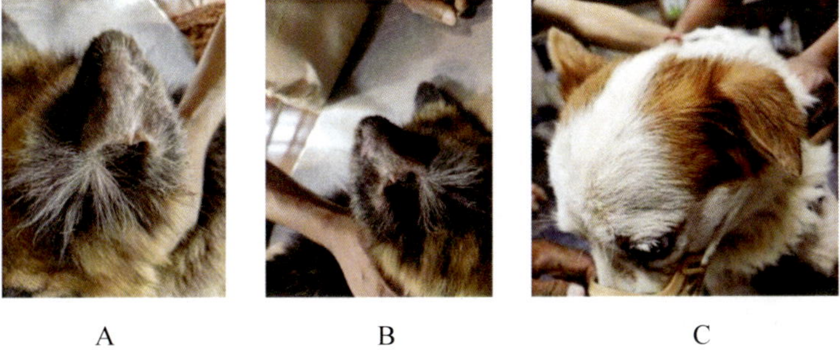

A B C

Fig. 28. Photographs of the German shepherd dog affected with aural hematoma and reduction in size of hematoma on Arnica and Hamamelis. A. Left ear pinna hematoma on day 0 (day of referral). B. Left ear pinna of the same German shepherd dog (at A) on day 21 post therapy with homeopathic Arnica and Hamamelis showing reduction in the size of the hematoma. C. Dog showing sign of dropped ear due to aural hematoma.

Clinical Management of non-suppurative wounds in animals with Homeopathic Calendula cream

J.P.Varshney (2024 d)

Ten cases of non-suppurative wounds (on head –Fig 29 A, interdigital space, limbs, abdomen)in dogs were treated with external application of homeopathic *Calendula* ointment once daily after cleaning the wound with sterile water. In these cases no parenteral antibiotic and /or antiseptic dressing was used . Observations were made daily on the progress of healing as well as development of suppuration if any and signs of infection. The healing in all cases continued with 1st intention without any sign of suppuration or infection. The wound contraction area increased daily. Basal body temperature in all cases remained within range (100.8 to 102.0 ^{0}F). Wounds in all 10 cases healed nicely though healing (Fig.29 B) time varied depending on the size of the wound.

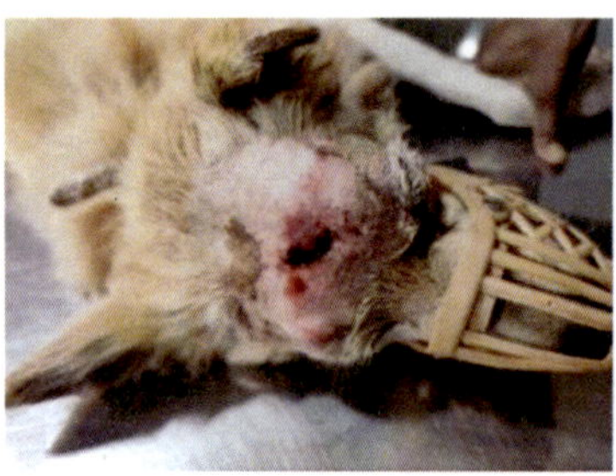

A

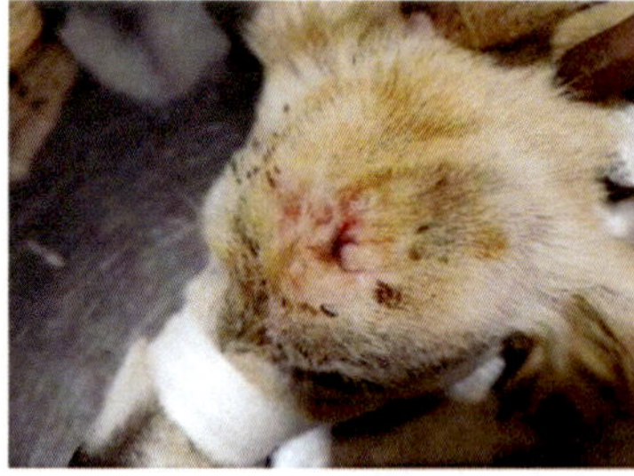

B

Fig. 29. Type of wounds in dogs treated with Calendula ointment. The piercing wound on head of the dog (A) at the initial stage. The wound was treated with homeopathic *Calendula* ointment without any antibiotic or modern antiseptic solution. The wound healed by 1st intention (no suppuration) in 10 days (B).

Clinical Management of Marked Epiphora with Euphrasia 10 % eye solution in kittens

J.P. Varshney (2024 e)

Twenty cases of marked epiphora in kittens (25 days to 60 day old) were referred at the hospital for diagnosis and treatment. History revealed that the epiphora was contagious as all kitten in the same house became affected. The clinical examination of the eye revealed almost bilateral marked serous eye discharge (epiphora) wetting the area around the eyes (Fig. 30 A), inflamed conjunctiva and varying degree of chemosis. Fluorescein eye stain test ruled out corneal ulceration in all cases. Schirmer tear test values varied from 20.0 to 25.0 mm/minute (STT value in healthy cats varies from 13.7 ± 4.6 to 15.7 ± 3.7

mm/minute) indicating increased tear production. Based on epidemiological and clinical picture , increased STT values and negative findings of fluorescein test, cases were diagnosed with marked epiphora associated with conjunctivitis akin to herpes infection in kitten. The cases were randomly divided into 3 groups. Group A consisting 10 kitten treated with homeopathic *Euphrasia* (10% eye drops) at the rate of one drop instilled into each eye four times daily; group B consisting 5 kitten treated with ciprofloxacin eye drops at the rate of one drop instilled in to each eye four times daily; and group C consisting of 5 kitten treated with sterile normal saline at the rate of one drop instilled into each eye four times daily. Initially the treatment was planned for one week. The outcome of treatment success was defined as no ocular discharge and returning of STT values with in normal range. Tearing reduced markedly (Fig.30 B) in kittens of group A with marked decrease in STT values (10 to 16 mm /minute). Whereas wetting of the hairs around eyes continued with no decrease in STT values (Group B 19.0-24.0 mm/minute ; Group C 22.0 to 26.0 mm/minute) in kittens of group B and C. Trial indicated that *Euphrasia* reduced reddening and tearing in the eyes of kittens.

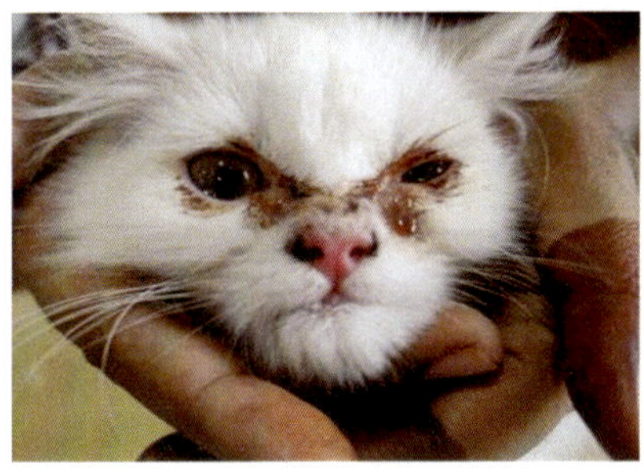

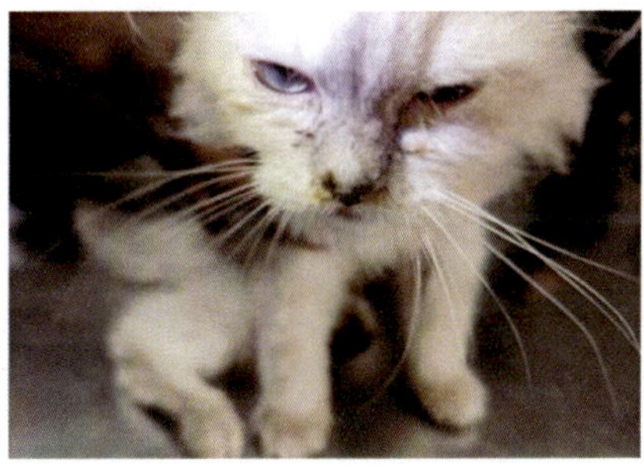

A B

Fig. 30 . Epiphora in kitten (A). Note marked tearing and wetting of the area near medial canthus. The same Kitten after 0ne week therapy with Euphrasia (B) showing marked reduction in tearing, no wetting near medial canthus.

Orexigenic Potential of Homopathic Alfalfa Q in Turtles

J.P. Varshney (2024 f)

Anorexia is a very common complaint in turtles . Its etiology is very wide ranging from dietetic abnormalities, husbandry errors, infections to diseases of internal organs.Post hibernation anorexia (i.e. the terrapin is warm and moving about but not eating) is more prevalent. Thirty apparently healthy turtles (body eight varying from 30 g to 4.0 kg, Male 22, female 08) with the complaint of anorexia for 4 to 14 days with no clinical signs (such as nasal discharge, bubbles at nostrils, foam at mouth commissures , soft shell, wound, erythema, ecto parasites or any swimming abnormality- Fig.31) and no radiographic evidence of any disease (such as respiratory tract abnormality, metabolic bone disease, enteroliths, uroliths, gaseous distension of stomach or intestines, or egg bound condition) were diagnosed with non-specific anorexia. All these turtles were active, responding to stimuli with normal swimming pattern . The anorectic turtles were randomly divided in to 2 groups of 15 anorectic turtle in each group. With the advice of proper husbandry practices, anorectic turtle of group A were treated with homeopathic *Alfalfa* Q tincture @ one drop given 4 times a day for a maximum period of 7 days . Where oral droppings were not feasible, it was advised to keep the turtle in water fortified @ 15 to 20 drops of Alfalfa Q per liter water. Turtles of group B were given placebo (water drops) in the manner similar to group A. Of 30, 22 turtles (73.3%) started eating their food in a period of 5 to 12 days. Revival of appetite was to the tune of 66.66% (10 out of 15) in group A and 20% (3 out 15) in group B with in a period of 7 days. It appears that Alfalfa has some potential in stimulating the appetite in turtle with non-specific anorexia.

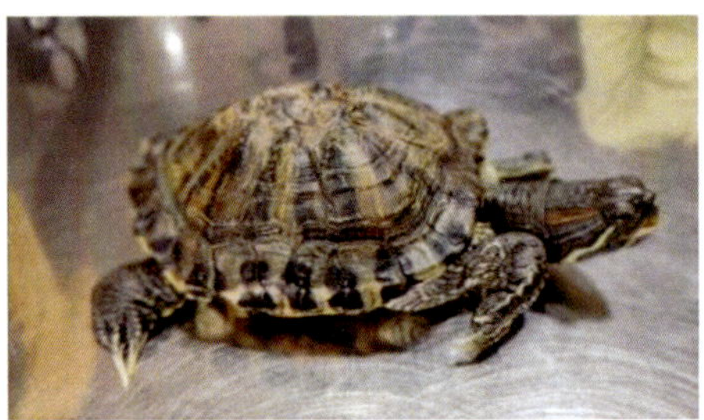

Fig. 31. Turtle with non-specific anorexia, showing no clinical and radiographic abnormality except no inclination for food.

Feline Icterus Owing to Hepatic Lipidosis Treated with Chelidonium 30 c

J.P. Varshney (2024 g)

Icterus (jaundice) is manifestation of hepatic and biliary diseases. It reflects higher bilirubin level. Jaundice in cats is a multi-etiology disease. Infection with feline leukemia virus or feline infectious peritonitis virus also predisposes cats to icterus. A fully vaccinated (Panleukopenia virus, Calci virus, Herpes virus and Rabies virus) 13 moth old female cat weighing 2.8 kg with the history of weight loss, yellowish eyes and inappetance for 5 days was referred for the diagnosis and treatment. Detail clinical examination revealed normal basal body temperature, vomiting, diarrhea, yellowish sclera (Fig.32 A) and mouth commissures, ptyalism, severe weakness and recumbency . Haemogram showed normal value of total leukocyte count (8500/ mm^3), severe anemia (total erythrocyte count 1.02 x10^6/mm^3, packed cell volume 10.3 %, hemoglobin 3.3

g/dl), thrombocytopenia (72000/mm^3), lymphocytosis (L 39%), Heinz body, and poikilocytosis. Biochemical investigation revealed an increased values of ALT (336.9 U/L), SAP (368.1 IU/L) , gamma- GT (30 U/L), trigylerides (190 mg/dl), total cholesterol (280 mg/dl) and bilirubin (total 17.38 mg/dl, direct 9.59 mg/dl, indirect 7.79 mg/dl); decreased values of total serum protein (4.2 g/dl), albumin (1.8 g/dl), blood urea nitrogen (6.2 mg/dl 8.0 mg/dl), blood glucose (68 mg/dl) and unaltered value of serum creatinine(1.0 mg/dl) . Abdominal radiography disclosed hepatomegaly . Homogenous hyperechoic hepatic parenchyma (Fig. 32 B) on abdominal survey ultrasonography was suggestive of hepatic cirrhosis or hepatic lipidosis. Clinical, biochemical , radiographic and ultrasonographic findings were suggestive of icterus owing to hepatic lipidosis. With the consent of the owner, the cat was treated with homeopathic drug *Chelidoinum* 30 c 2drops four times daily along with intravenous amino acid and glucose therapy (@ 60 ml /kg body weight IV fortified with vitamin B complex 0.2 ml). Improvement in general condition began on day 3rd. On resumption of oral feeding on 6th day parenteral fluid therapy was stopped. The cat was much comfortable and active. Laboratory investigation on day 14th showed marked improvement (increase in total erythrocyte count 2.12 x10 ^{6}/mm^3, packed cell volume 18.3 %, hemoglobin 6.3 g/dl , thrombocyte count 230,000/mm^3 , total serum proteins 5.1 g/dl, albumin 2.8 g/dl , BUN 10 mg/dl, glucose 82 mg/dl :and decrease in lymphocyte count 26 % , a few Heinz body, reduced poikilocytosis , ALT 186.4 U/L, SAP 201.3 IU/L , gamma- GT 22 U/L , trigylerides 172 mg/dl, total cholesterol 220 mg/dl , bilirubin total 9.8 mg/dl, direct 5.7 mg/dl, indirect 4.1 mg/dl and no changes in serum creatinine 1.0 mg/dl). The dose of *Chelidonium* was reduced to two times a day and continued for another two weeks. The cat was eating its normal food and was more active and vigorous with normal colored sclara and mucus membranes. It appears that *Chelidonium* 30 c with supportive therapy showed promising results in the management of icteric cat with hepatic lipidosis.

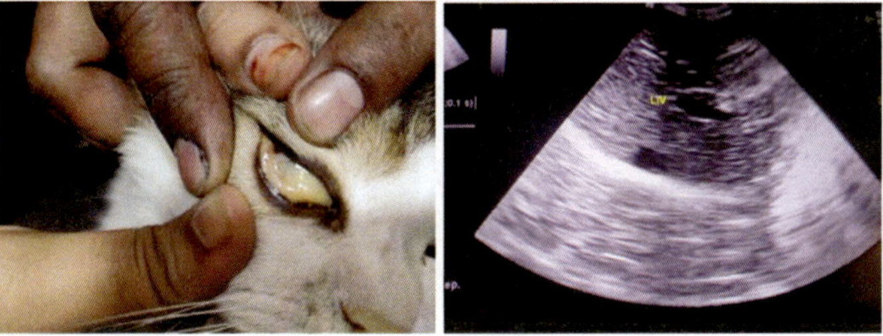

A B

Fig. 32. Cat suffering from lipidosis is showing icteric sclera (A) and its abdominal ultrasound is showing hyperechoic hepatic parenchyma (B).

Clinical Management of Neck Trauma in a kitten with Homeopathic Drugs.

J.P. Varshney (2024 h)

A four month old female kitten (2.450 kg) was referred at the hospital with the history of traumatic injury on the neck (inflicted by a dog who caught the kitten by neck 40 minutes before) , nasal and oral bleeding, neck and head turned to the left , seizures , inability to keep head and neck in normal aligned position, open mouth breathing and recumbency (Fig. 33 A and 33 B). Clinical examination at the time of referral revealed nasal and buccal bleeding; dyspnea; mouth open; salivation; swelling in neck region; elicitation of pain, seizures and paddling (Fig.33 B) on cervical palpation; inability to keep neck and head in straight alignment leading to turning of neck and head on left side (concavity on left and convexity on right side of neck); and increased temperature (104.2^{0}F) . Radiographic examination (Fig. 33 C) revealed neither any detectable abnormality of cervical boney architecture nor any lung pathology . Nasal examination revealed bilateral bleeding making the respiration difficult. Ear examination revealed no fluid/ blood. Functional evaluation of cranial nerve VIII was normal. Electrocardiogram was within normal range. Based on history, symptoms , physical , radiographic and electrocardiographic evaluations, the kitten was diagnosed with neck trauma. The treatment was initiated with *Arnica* 30c and *Hamamelis* 30c one drop each (keeping 15 minutes gap between both medicines) twice , ice fomentation on nasal area and wet cloth sponging on head when temperature increases after seizures and keeping the neck and head on pillow to keep head and neck aligned (Fig. 33 D) on the day of 1st day. The owner was advised to give oral rehydrating solution by dropper frequently. Evaluation on next day (2nd day) revealed traces of occasional oral and nasal bleeding , anorexia , recumbency and palpation of neck evoked pain and convulsions leading to increase in body temperature. Therapy given on 1st day was continued on 2nd day. On day 3rd there was no bleeding, stabilized respiration. *Hamamelis* was stopped , *Arnica* was continued and *Hypericum* 200 c one drop thrice daily was added. On day 4th the kitten was quite comfortable started recognizing the owner, raising head and attempting to stand, neck palpation did not elicit seizures but the cat was anorectic. *Arnica* and *Hypericum* were continued and the kitten was given 100 ml Ringer's lactate parenterally. On day 5th the kitten raised head , stood up (Fig. 33 E) and took few steps, but remained ataxic and anorectic. Treatment given on 4th day was repeated. On 6th day the kitten started standing (Fig.33 F) , moving and aligning head and neck (Fig. 33 G), without seizure and pain on palpation of neck but appetite was still poor. *Hypericum* and *Arnica* was stopped and *Alfalfa* Q 1-2 drop in water was advised twice daily till resumption of appetite. On day 8th the cat was fully active keeping neck and head aligned with no pain on neck palpation, no seizures and started taking her usual food (Fig. 33 H) . *Arnica* was selected for its symptoms of injury (due to catching by dog, vertigo type symptoms, nasal and buccal injury, unconsciousness and neck pain on palpation. Symptoms of hemorrhage from nose, buccal cavity were matching with *Hamamelis virginica. Hypericum* matched with the symptoms of injuries to the nerves, tremors or seizures after injury and injured nerves from animal bite (the kitten neck was caught in mouth by the dog).Selection of *Alfalfa* matched with the symptom of impaired appetite. The kitten fully recovered from traumatic neck injury due to dog within 8 days with the homeopathic treatment adopted.

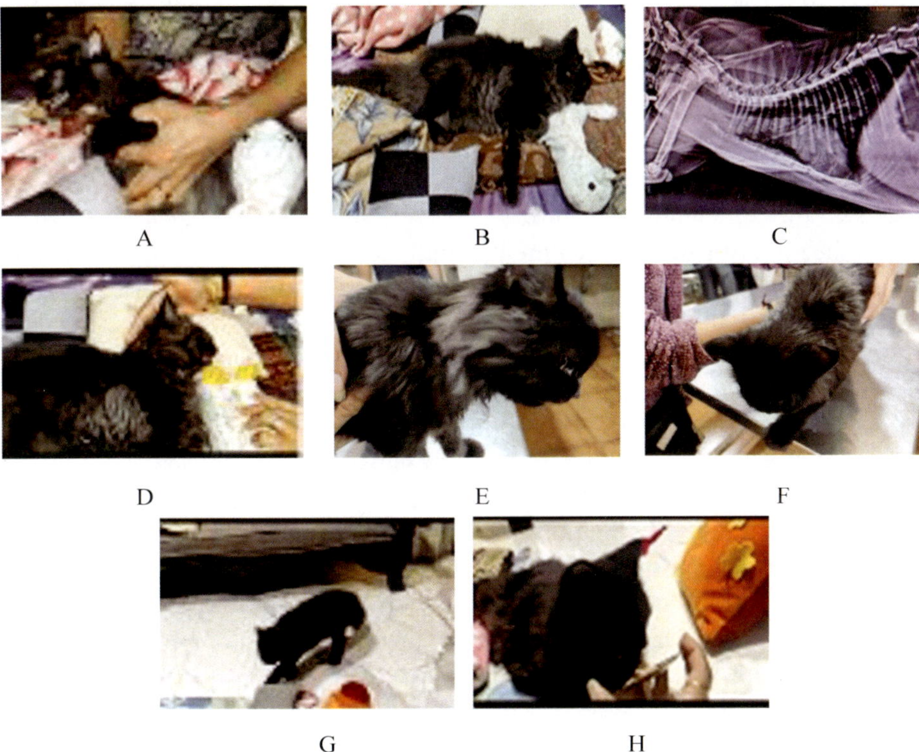

Fig. 33. Cat with neck trauma in different clinical stages. A. and B. showing nasal and oral bleeding, neck and head turned to the left , seizures , inability to keep head and neck in normal aligned position, open mouth breathing and recumbency. C, Radiographic examination revealing neither any detectable abnormality of cervical boney architecture nor any lung pathology. D. neck and head on pillow to keep head and neck aligned.E. the kitten raised head and tried to get up. F.Kitten standing.G. Kitten walking with aligned head and neck normally. H. Kitten started taking her food.

Clinical Management of Chronic Cases of Pseudomonas Otitis in Dogs with Homeopathic combination Remedy

J.P.Varshney (2024 i)

Pseudomonas aeruginosa is ubiquitous in environment but uncommon inhabitant of ear canal of dogs. It is a most common opportunistic pathogen in chronic otitis.

The infection is proliferated in moist anaerobic environment producing exotoxins and polysaccharide slime layer that protects it from host immune system, moderate to high level of multiple drug resistance to commonly used antibiotics by efflux pumps and rapid mutation make it difficult to treat the infection completely. Six chronic cases of otitis media/otitis interna refractory to marbofloxacin were selected with homeopathic treatment with the informed consent of the owners. The clinical manifestations were characterized by head shaking, ear scratching and pain on manipulation of pinna, excessive aural discharge , and ulcerated ears filled with malodorous exudates (Fig.34 A) . Cytological and cultural examinations of ear swabs revealed the preponderance of Gram negative bacilli (Fig.34 B). Based on oxidase and other biochemical reaction the organism was identified as *Pseudomonas aeruginosa.* The recurrence of otitis despite treatment with three –four antibiotics in succession during last few months made the owners frustrated. With their informed consent of the owners, homeopathic treatment was instituted with biweekly ear flushing (5% povidone iodine solution- Fig 34 C) and a homeopathic combination remedy consisting of *Mercurius sol.*30 c, *Hepar sulph* 30c, *Silicea* 30 c and *Pulsatilla* 30 c (mixed in equal proportion)given @ 4drops orally four times daily initially for seven days. Then twice daily till improvement or a period of 8 weeks whichever is earlier. *Merc.sol , Hepar sulph, Silicea and Pulsatilla* were selected for their indications in chronic ear infection, foetid ear discharge with ear pain, suppurative processes and thick foetid discharge respectively. Out of six cases only one case showed clinical and bacteriological recovery at the end of 8th week. Three cases showed remarkable reduction in ear discharge and ear shaking but no bacteriological clearance at the end of 8th week. In other two cases there was fluctuation in head shaking and in the amount of ear discharge with persistence of *Pseudomonas* at the end of 8th week.

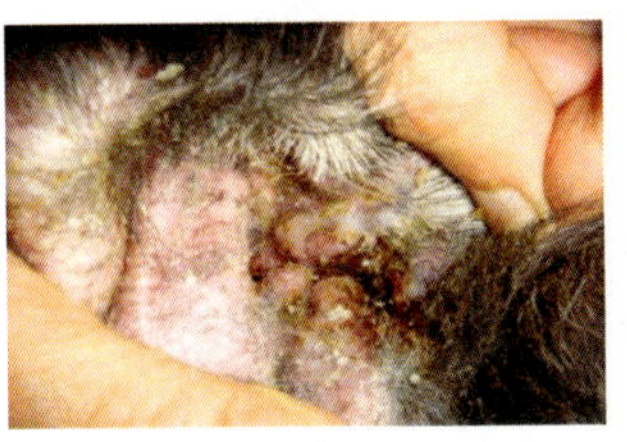
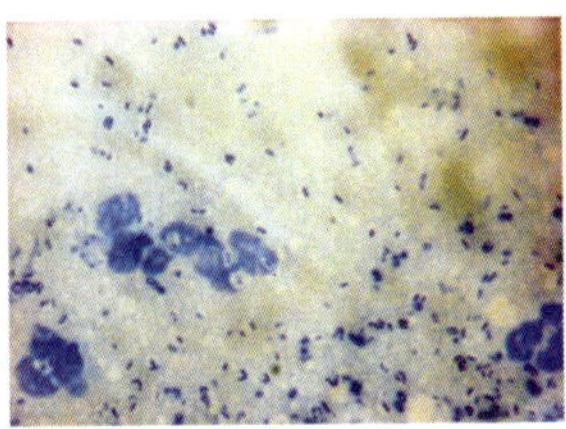
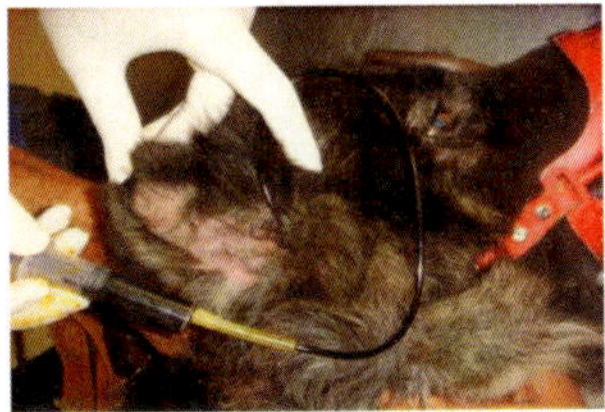

A B C

Fig. 34. Otitis media in dog. A. showing excessive aural discharge, and ulcerated ears filled with malodorous exudates. B. Cytological examinations of ear swabs revealed the preponderance of Gram negative bacilli. Based on oxidase and other biochemical reaction the organism was identified as *Pseudomonas aeruginosa***.** C. Ear flushing with 5% povidone iodine solution.

Clinical Management of Corneal Ulcers in a Dog with Silica terra 30c and Euphrasia 10 % eye solution

J.P. Varshney (2024 j)

Corneal ulcer is one of the most common eye disease in dog that can lead to vision loss. Corneal ulcer, also known as ulcerative keratitis, is an inflammation of cornea associated with loss of the corneal epithelium caused by any condition (traumatic or non-traumatic) that damages the corneal epithelium or stroma. A 10- year-old intact male Lhasa Apso weighing10.0 kg (named Zuzu), was referred at the hospital on 4th May,24 with the main complaint of tearing and photophobia in the both eyes for days .The treatment adopted with antibiotics (advised by local vet) remained ineffective. Clinical examination revealed a good overall condition, normal heart and respiratory rates and normal temperature (102.2°F). Ophthalmic examination revealed lesions in both eyes characterized by corneal edema (Fig.35 A) conjunctival and scleral hyperemia (Fig.35 B), perforated cornea (Fig.35 D), accompanied by epiphora, photophobia, blepharospasm, pain, frequent closing the eyes, pawing at eyes, and rubbing face. A fluorescein test (Fig. 35C) , performed in both eye, was positive, showing rupture of the corneal epithelium and represented by a considerable erosive process (Figure35 D) leading to the diagnosis of deep corneal ulcer of traumatic origin. The treatment was initiated with homeopathic *Euphrasi*a eye drops (10% instilled three times a day), *Arnica* 30 c (2-3 drops twice daily for 3 days initially) and *Silica terra* 30c (2-3 drops thrice daily for ten days followed by twice daily till recovery). On 10th day (1st post therapeutic visit) there was marked reduction in pain, epiphora, scleral and conjunctival hyperemia and pawing at eyes. The treatment was continued except that frequency of dosing of *Silica* was reduced to twice daily. The dog visited hospital again after 42 days of therapy with no epiphora, no pawing at eyes, no pain, no conjunctival and scleral hyperemia, no photophobia and no mark of corneal perforation. The healing and regeneration of affected corneal epithelium was complete (Fig.35 E) as there was no retention of fluorescein dye. The homeopathic drugs chosen were based on anato-mopathological similarities. *Silica terra* is considered as a polycrest medicine and most appropriate in cases with perforating /sloughing corneal ulcers, confused vision, aversion to light , sharp eye pain . *Euphrasia* is indicated for balancing the ophthalmic environment and *Arnica* in indicated in cases of injury.

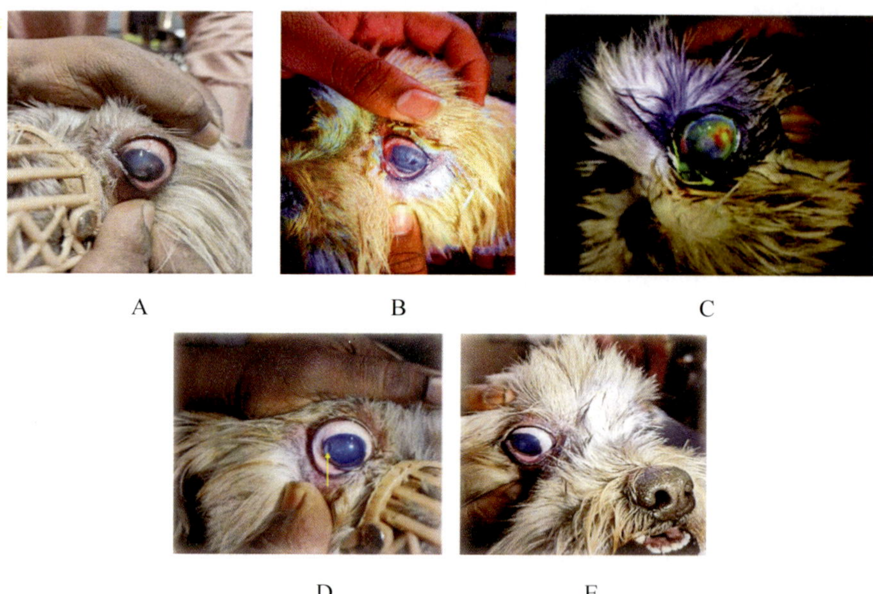

Fig. 35. Corneal Ulcers and edema in a Lhasa Apso 10 year old male dog treated with *Silica* and *Euphrasia*.A. Corneal edema. B. Scleral hyperemia .C.Positive fluorescein test showing rupture of the corneal epithelium confirming corneal ulcer.D. Showing ulceration in the right eye (A marked with yellow arrow) before treatment at the time of referral. E. Showing healed up ulcer and complete marked improvement in the right eye after forty two days of therpay with *Silica* 30c 2 drops orally twice daily along with eye instilation of 10% *Euphrasia* eye drops.

Clinical Management of Seborrhea sicca in a Dog with Sulphur 30c

J.P. Varshney (2024 k)

Seborrhea is a common skin disease in dog characterized by excessive keratinization of epidermal layer of the skin often secondary to infection or inflammation. Primary seborrhea is inherited skin disease seen in some breeds of dogs (American Cocker Spaniels, English Springer Spaniels, Basset Hounds, West Highland White Terriers, Dachshunds, Labrador and Golden Retrievers, and German Shepherd). While secondary seborrhea is a symptom of underlying disease (inflammation, infection or hormonal imbalance). A four-year-old non-descript dog weighing 16.5 kg was referred at the hospital with the complaint of dandruff lasting for 5-6 months refractory to routine treatment. Detailed clinical examination at referral revealed slim body, excessive dry scaling and crusting on the back (Fig.36 A), no foul smell from body , no marked itching, dry and hard hairs and skin, and normal appetite. Flea combing test and skin scrapings were negative ruling out fleas and mange mite infestation. Acetate tape smear showed no *Malassezia* but few Gram +ve cocci. Laboratory investigations revealed normal levels of thyroid (fT3 2.94 pg/ml, fT4 1.01 ng/dl) and cortisol (1.32μg/dl) hormones ruling out hormonal etiology of the seborrhea. Based on the presence of excessive dry scales on the back, no marked irritation, absence of mange mites (Scabies and Demodex) and fleas, and normal levels of thyroid and cortisol, the dog was diagnosed with *Seborrhea sicca*. With the informed consent of the owner, the treatment was initiated with homeopathic *Sulphur* 30c (2-3 drops twice daily for two weeks then once daily till complete absence of scaling) with weekly evaluation. There was no appreciable response on first weekly visit but decrease in scaling became apparent on 2nd weekly visit. On 5th weekly visit there was complete absence of dry scales and crusting on back (Fig.36 B) indicating that homeopathic *Sulphur* 30c has great potential in the management of secondary *Seborrhea sicca* in dogs. The total cost of treatment was around rupees thirty.

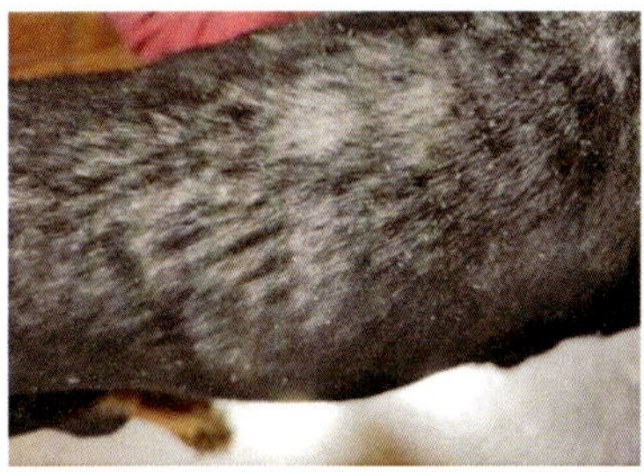

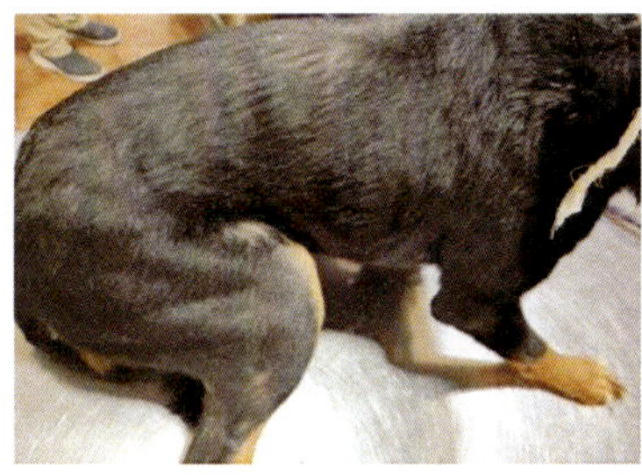

A B

Fig. 36. Seborrhoea in a four year old non-descript dog. It is clinically characterized by excessive dry scaling and crusting on the back (A), no foul smell from body, no marked itching, dry and hard hairs and skin, and normal appetite.The dog was negative for ticks, mange mites and malassazia and had normal values of thyroid and cortisol levels. Treatment with Sulphur 30 c led to complete recovery in 35 days (B).

Experimental Studies

Evaluation of the Efficacy of A Homeo-complex in Prevention of Cholesterol -cholic Acid Induced Cholelithiasis in Mice model

B.Bandyopadhyay, J.P. Varshney and O.P. Paliwal (2007)

The present investigation was undertaken to evaluate the efficacy of a homeocomplex (consisting of *Andrographis panniculata* 1x, *Carica P* 2x, *Chelidonium* 1x, *Myrica ceri* 1x and *Chionanthus* 1x in equal proportion 0.4% V/V) in prevention of cholesterol cholic acid induced choletiths in mice. Feeding of cholesterol (1%) and cholic acid (0.5%) enriched diet not only induced choleliths (Fig.37) but also damaged the liver in mice. Formation of choleliths could not be prevented completely by concurrent use of the homeocomplex or ursodeoxycholic acid (UDCA). Nevertheless, decrease in elevated levels of ALT, SAP, gamma-GT, total and direct bilirubin, cholesterol and triglyceride indicated hepato protective potential as well as lipid lowering ability of the homeo-complex. UDCA showed better results than the homeo-complex in preventing formation of choleliths, nevertheless, it also did not prove to be 100% efficacious.

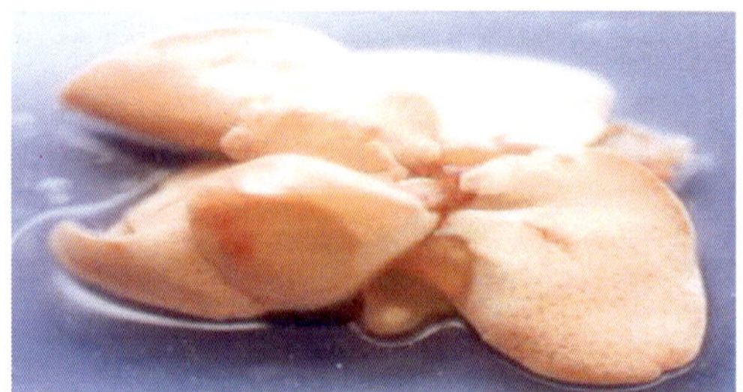

Fig. 37. Highly enlarged liver and distinct gall stone is the gall bladder of a mice fed on lithogenic diet.

Evaluation of Hypolipidaemic and Hepatoprotective Efficacy of a Homeo-complex in Mice Fed on Cholesterol Enriched Diet

S. Bandyopadhyay, J.P. Varshney and Ghosh, M.K. (2007)

An experimental study on evaluation of hypolipidaemic and hepatoprotective efficacy of a homeo-complex (consisting of *Andrographis paniculata* 1 x, *Carica P.* 2 x, *Chelidonium majus* 1 x, *Myrica ceri* 1 x, and *Chionanthus* 1 x, 0.4% each v/v) in mice model was conducted . Three months feeding on cholesterol (1%)-cholic acid (0.5%) enriched diet induced choleliths in mice with higher serum cholesterol (357.90 ± 28.25 mg/dl), low density lipo-protein (284.83 ± 33.5 mg/dl), triglycerides (87.21 ± 2.28 mg/dl), ALT (103.667 ±

0.479 U/L), Alkaline phosphatase (119.808 ± 7.476 U/L) and gamma-GT (15.348 ± 3.039 U/L) in gr. B. With simultaneous administration of the homeo-complex in gr-C mice on the same cholesterol-cholic acid enriched diet, serum cholesterol (281.86 ± 26.75 mg/dl), low density lipo-protein (207.32 ± 5.78 mg/dl), triglycerides (53.34 ± 4.71 mg/dl), ALT (71.83 ± 9.06 U/L), Alkaline phosphatase (88.63 ± 13.92 U/L) and g-GT (10.17 ± 0.88 U/L) levels were significantly ($P<0.01$) low as compared to diseased control (gr.B) group. From the present study it appears that the homeo-complex seems to have hypolipidaemic and hepatoprotective potential.

Evaluation of hepatoprotective efficacy of homeopathic drugs in carbon tetrachloride induced hepatopathy in rats – An experimental study

S.Soja Saghar, J.P. Varshney and O.P. Paliwal (2007)

The present investigation was conducted to evaluate the hepatoprotective efficacy of homeopathic formulations in carbon tetrachloride induced hepatopathy in rats. Carbon tetrachloride induced hepato toxicity in rats was characterized by jaundice, weakness and reduced feed intake; marked elevation of activities of serum enzymes (ALT-48.00 ± 8.62 U/L, gamma -GT-27.60 ± 9.98 U/L, SAP –62.77 ± 7.29 U/L), increased serum bilirubin (total – 1.85 ± 0.28 mg/dl and direct – 0.45 ± 0.10 mg/dl), decreased serum total protein (5.94 ± 0.62 g/dl), albumin (2.61 ± 0.40 g/dl) and blood glucose (73.80 ± 13.40 mg/dl); increased liver: body weight ratio; and hydropic degeneration and vacuolation in the liver. Medication with homeopathic formulation containing *Andrographis paniculata, Carica P, Chelidornium majus, Myrica ceri, Chionanthus* in syrup base and in pill form could keep these indices near normal during the observation period of 8 weeks and compared well with a reference herbal drug Silymarin indicating hepatoprotective potential of the homeopathic combination remedies.

Anti-inflammatory Activity of a Homeo- complex in Carrageenan Induced Hindpaw Odema in Rats

J.P. Varshney, S.K. Tandon and S.P. Dudhgaonkar (2007)

An experimental study on anti-inflammatory activity of a homeo-complex (consisting of *Phytolacca* 200C, *Calcarea fluorica* 200C, *Silicia* 30C, *Belladonna* 30C, *Bryonia* 30C, *Arnica* 30C, *Conium* 30C and I*pecacuanha* 30C) was conducted in rat model. Interplanter injection of carrageenan (100 µl,1.0% suspension w/v) in rat resulted in an increase in hind paw volume (oedema) characterized by a rapid 'early' phase (upto 3h) response (50.28 to 64.77% increase in paw volume in all groups) followed by a more sustained late phase (3-7 h) response (75.54 to 77.24% increase in paw volume) in rats of disease control group A. Oral administration of 0.2 ml aqueous solution (10 pills in 1 ml distilled water) of the homeo complex beginning at 30 min. interval for three times at 3 h post carrageenan injection reduced the increased paw volume significantly ($P<0.05-0.01$) with a mean per cent inhibition of 6.30 at 5 h, 12.6 at 7 h and 20.03 at 10 h. while reduction in per cent oedema volume (17.95) in rats of gr.A was evident only at 10 h. It is quite evident from the present study that the homeocomplex possesses anti inflammatory activity.

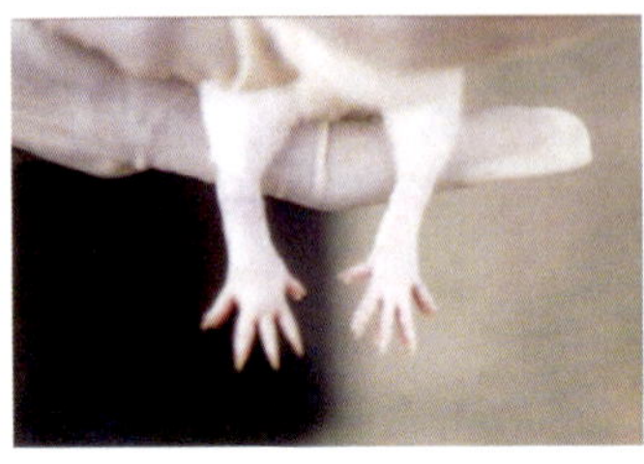

Fig. 38. Physical changes in right hind paw of a rat of group A at 10 h post carrageenan injection.

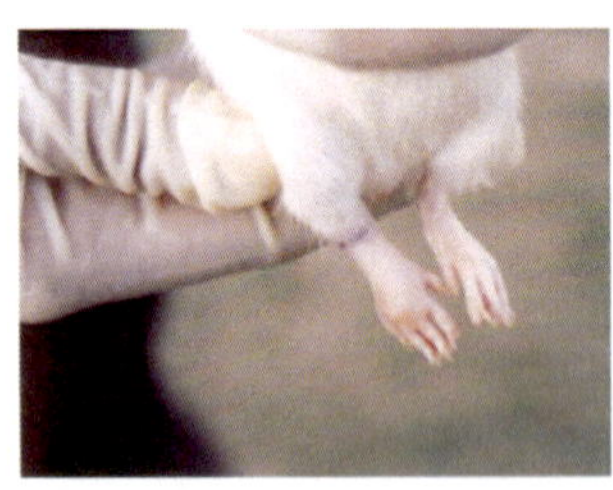

Fig. 39. Physical changes in right hind paw of a rat of group B (Treated with aspirin) at 10 h post carrageenan injection.

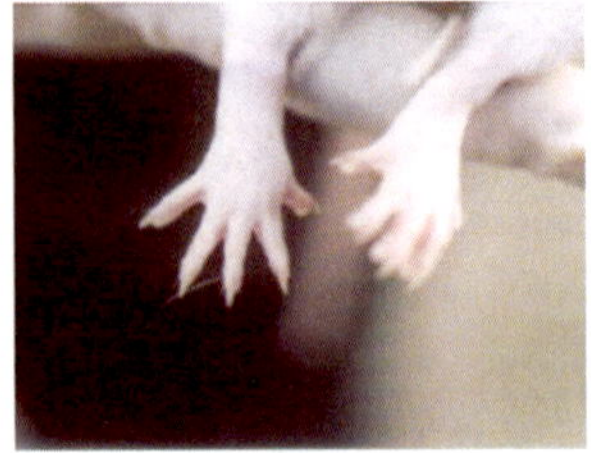

Fig. 40. Physical changes in right hind paw of a rat of group-C (treated with Homeo complex VT-6) at 10 h. post carrageenan injection.

Evaluation of Anti-pyretic Efficacy of Homeopathic Drugs in Brewer's Yeast Induced Pyrexia

J.P. Varshney, S.K. Tandon and A.S. Bhat (2007)

An experimental controlled study on antipyretic efficacy of homeopathic drugs (*Arsenic album* 30C alone, and a homeo-complex consisting of *Aconite* 30C, *Arsenic alb*. 30 C, *Belladonna* 30C, *Ferrum phos* 30C and *Kali mur* 30C, in equal proportions), keeping healthy, disease and an allopathic drug controls, was conducted. Subcutaneous injection of Brewer's yeast (20% suspension) @ 10 ml Kg^{-1} produced pyrexia in 18 hrs. Oral administration of 0.2ml aqueous sol. of *Arsenic album* (Group D) and a homeo-complex (Group C) three times at 15 min. interval beginning at 18 h post Brewer's yeast injection failed to reduce pyrexia and rectal temperature at 19, 21, 23, and 25th hours post

Brewer's yeast injection remained elevated as compared to 0 hr values and to that of healthy controls. While paracetamol (group E) could significantly reverse the increase in temperature at 19 and 21 hours but temperature again increased at 23 and 25-h post Brewer's yeast injection.It is evident from the experiment that neither homeo *Arsenic album* alone nor a homeo-complex showed antipyretic efficacy in Brewer's yeast induced pyrexia in mice. Even paracetamol failed to reduce pyrexia completely during whole experimental period.

Homeopathy Treatment of Malassezia pachydermatis in vitro

T.A.R. Goncalves, J.R.de. úlia Roriz de Oliveira, E.Perrone, S.D.A. Coutinho and L.V. Bonamin (2022).

A common clinical occurrence in dogs is otitis externa caused by excessive growth of yeasts *Malassezia pachydermatis*, which can become chronic after wrong treatments, in which microbial resistance can occur. Homeopathic remedies can be considered a successful alternative, selecting the medicine through the similitude principle. Herein, 50 µL of a 1:1000 dilution of *Malassezia pachydermatis* suspension at 0.5 McFarland scale was used to seed the yeast into Sabouraud dextrose agar plates using a Drigalski spreader to proceed with colony unit counting. Before being seeded, the yeast suspensions were treated with 1% of different homeopathic treatments previously selected from a pilot study, which means *Sulphur* 6cH, *Dolichos pruriens* 6cH, and *Kali carbonicum* 6cH, being water, and succussed water used as controls. For comparison, a set of Sabouraud dextrose agar plates containing 1% Tween 80 was seeded in parallel. The treatments were made blind and evaluated in triplicate. Contaminated cultures were withdrawn. The number of colonies per plate was assessed, and smears were made from the cultures to classify yeast growth according to cytomorphology on ImageJ® software. The preliminary results show no significant effect of all tested medicines compared to the controls. High data variability was also observed, mainly in those cultures whose medium was prepared with Twin 80. In conclusion, at this point of the study, no evidence of the effects of the studied medicines on *Malassezia pachydermatis* growth in vitro could be identified.

References and Literature Reviewed

Ajay Kumar and Varshney, J.P. (2005). A preliminary study on antihaemorrhagic efficacy of a homeo-complex in the management of hemorrhagic crisis in dogs. Natn. Seminar Homeopathic medicine Plant Animals and Fishes, Thrissur, 5-6th February,05,p.79.

Ajay Kumar and Varshney,J.P. (2007).Hepatotrophic potential of a Homeo-complex in the management of secondary hepatopathy associated with a mixed infection of E.canis and B.gibsoni in Dogs. In: Research Findings. Homeopathic Bioefficacy and Management of

Animal Health. Varshney, J.P. and Swaminarayan, S (eds). Sintex International Limited, Kalol, pp.81-85.

Bandyopadhyay, S. , Varshney, J.P. and Paliwal, O.P.(2007).Evaluation of the Efficacy of A Homeo-complex in Prevention of Cholesterol –cholicAcid Induced Cholelithiasis in Mice model. In: Research Findings. Homeopathic Bioefficacy and Management of Animal Health. Varshney, J.P. and Swaminarayan, S (eds). Sintex International Limited, Kalol, pp.74-80.

Bandyopadhyay,S. , Varshney,J.P. and Ghosh, M.K. (2007). Evaluation of hypolipidemic and hepatoprotective efficacy of a homeopathic complex in mice fed on cholesterol enriched diet. Indian J.Vet.Med.27:142-143.

Bandyopadhyay, S. and Varshney,J.P.(2008). Clinicotherapeutic management of hepatitis associated with Gallbladder sludge in a Dog. Intas Polivet 9 : 180-182.

Bandyopathyay, S., Varshney,J.P., Hoque,H., Swarup,D., Biswas, T.K., Bora, M. and Ghosh, M.K. (2010).Homeopathic treatment of cholecystitis disorders in dogs. Indian Vet.J. 2010 ; 981-983.

Changkija, B. and Varshney, J.P. (2005). Effect of Abies nigra on heart rate and rhythm in tachycardimic dogs- A case study. International Homeopathic Conference, Toronto, Canada, October 22-23, 05.

Changkija, B. and Varshney, J.P. (2007). Clinical Management of Bradycardia in a Non-Descript Dog with Abies nigra. In: Research Findings.Homeopathic Bioefficacy and Management of Animal Health. Varshney, J.P. and Swaminarayan, S (eds). Sintex International Limited, Kalol, pp.167-170.

Chaudhuri,S, and Varshney,J.P.(2007a). Clinical mangement of babesiosis in dogs with homeopathic Crotalus horridus 200c. Homeopathy 96:90-94.

Chaudhuri ,S. and Varshney,J.P.(2007b).Clinical management of anaemia associated with babesiosis in dogs with Trinitrotoluenum 200c. Homeopathic Links Autumn 20:162-164. @ Sonntag Verlog in MVS,Medizinverlage GmbH & Co. KG

Choudhury,B.K. ,Choudhury, S.,Meher, J., Dash,M., Bagh,S. ,Behera,B.K. and Ratha,S.(2024). Clinical Management of Pustular Dermatitis in Goats with Homeopathic Drugs (personal communication). Email: bimal.vet@gmail.com

Goncalves, T.A.R., úlia Roriz de Oliveira, J.R.de,Perrone,E.,Coutinho, S.D.A. and Bonamin,L.V. (2022). Homeopathy Treatment of Malassezia pachydermatis in vitro. International J. High Dilution Research - ISSN 1982-6206, 21(2), 10–10. https://doi.org/10.51910/ijhdr.v21i2.1206.

Gopinathan, A., Pawde, A.M. and Singh, K. (2007).Effect of Calendula officinalisin Burn Wounds f Calves and Heifers. In: Research Findings.Homeopathic Bioefficacy and Management of Animal Health. Varshney, J.P. and Swaminarayan, S (eds). Sintex International Limited, Kalol, pp.175-182.

Harendra Kumar,Srivastava,S.K.,Yadav, M.C. and Varshney, J.P (2003). Management of post-partum anestrus in dairy animals with a homeopathic combination remedy.Nat.Symp. Challenges Strategies Sust.Anim.Prod. in Mountains, Palampur, 14th-15th April,2003.

Harendra Kumar, S.K.Srivastava, M.C.Yadav and J.P.Varshney (2004). Management of post partum anestrus in dairy animals with a homeopathic combination remedy. Indian J.Anim.Sci.74:739-740.

Hwang,,H.K., Yang,H.G.,Kim,M.S. and Kim,N.S (2011). The effect of the pulsatilla 30C as homeopathy for ophthalmic diseases with concomitant separation anxiety J Vet Clin 2011; 28(1): 173-178.

Raj Kumar, R.,Srivastava,S.K., Yadav,M.C., Harendra Kumar, Varshney ,V.P.and Varshney, J.P. (2004).Effect of homeopathic combination remedy on estrus induction and hormonal profile in anestrus cows. XX Annual Convention of ISSAR and National Symposium, Durg, 14th –16th Dec.,2004, pp 39-40.

Raj Kumar, R., Srivastava, S.K., Yadav, M.C., Varshney,V.P., Varshney,J.P. andKumar,H. (2006).Effect of a Homeopathic complex on oestrus induction and hormonal profile in anoestrus cows. Homeopathy 95:131-135.

Raj, P.A.A., Pavulraj, S., Kumar, M.A., Sangeetha, S., Shamugapriya, R.and Sabithabanu,S. (2020).Therapeutic evaluation of homeopathic treatment for canine oral papillomatosis, Veterinary World, 13:206-213.

Ram Naresh, Varshney,J.P. and Mukherjee, Reena (2002). Management of udder affections with homeopathic formulation – a preliminary trial. 10th International Congress AAAP, NewDelhi, 23rd-27th September, 2002.

Ram Naresh and Varshney,J.P.(2004). Management of nonspecific diarrhoea syndrome in calves with a homeopathic combination remedy. Indian J.Vet.Med.24:58

Ram Naresh and Varshney,J.P. (2005). Management of bovine udder affections with a combination therapy. Homeopathic Links Summer 18:1 04-106. @ Sonntag Verlog in MVS,Medizinverlage GmbH & Co. KG

Risheen, G. D, Walwadker, K.K., Mishra,K.k. and Shrivastava, S. (2022). Therapeutic efficacy of homeopathy (Crotalus horridus) and allopathy (Doxycycline) drugs in Canine Ehrlichiosis. The Pharma Innovation J. SP-11(3): 253-256.

Saghar, Soja, S., Varshney, J.P. and Paliwal,O.P.(2007).Evaluation of hepatoprotective efficacy of homeopathic drugs in carbon tetrachloride induced hepatopathy in rats – An experimental study. In: Research Findings. Homeopathic Bioefficacy and Management of Animal Health. Varshney, J.P and Swaminarayan, S. (eds). Sintex International Limited, Kalol, pp.43-54.

Saghar, Soja, S., Varshney, J.P. and Hoque, M. (2007). Evaluation of Hepatoprotective Efficacy of a Homeo-complex in Dogs with Hepatopathy. In: Research Findings. Homeopathic Bioefficacy and Management of Animal Health. Varshney, J.P.and Swaminarayan, S (eds). Sintex International Limited, Kalol, pp.64-73.

Scardoeli , B.,Narita,F.B., Pinheiro, S.R., Ancken,A von and Cidéli de Paula Coelho,C.de P. (2021).Homeopathic Treatment of Trauma, Abscess and Papillomatosis in Trachemys dorbigni.Int.J.High Dilution Resch. ISSN 1982-6206, 18(02), 04–04. https://doi.org/10.51910/ijhdr.v18i02.985.

Scott, D.W., Miller,W.H. Jr., Senter, D.A., Cook,C.P., Edward Kirker,J. and Cobb, S.M.(2002). Treatment of canine atopic dermatitis with a commercial homeopathic remedy: A single-blinded, placebo-controlled study. Can Vet J. 2002 Aug; 43(8): 601–603.

Somvanshi, R. (2007). Preliminary observations on efficacy of homeopathic medicines in firld cases of boveine hematuria. In: Research Findings. Homeopathic Bioefficacy and Management of Animal Health. Varshney, J.P. and Swaminarayan, S. (eds). Sintex International Limited, Kalol. pp 110-111.

Somvanshi, R. and Sharma, R.D. (2007).Therapeutic Management of Cutaneous Warts in A Heifer By Thuja .In: Research Findings. Homeopathic Bioefficacy and Management of Animal Health. Varshney, J.P. and Swaminarayan, S. (eds). Sintex International Limited, Kalol. pp 150-151.

Varshney , J.P.(2003).Evaluation of a homeopathic combination remedy in the management of canine viral gastroenteritis simulating to parvo. Natn. Symp. Focussing Need Develop New Diag.Therap.Prev.ApproachesDeal Disorders farm Comp.Anims. Anand, 7th-9th February,2003.

Varshney, J.P. and Ajay Kumar (2003). Management of pyrexia syndrome with a homeopathic combination remedy. 14th International Homeopathic Congress. 17th -19th October,2003, New Delhi, India.

Varshney , J.P. and Ram Naresh (2003). Management of udder affections of Indian buffaloes with a homeopathic combination remedy. 4th AsianBuffalo Congress, NewDelhi, 25th-28th February,2003.

Varshney, J.P. (2004). Management of pyrexia in animals with homeopathic drug. World Herbo Expo-2004, Bhopal, 12th-14th January,2004.

Varshney, J.P. and Ajay Kumar (2004). Clnical management of epilepsy in dogs with homeopathic drugs. Natn.Symp.Latest Approaches Biotech.Tools Hlth.Manage.Farm Comp.Anims.,Izatnagar, 11th-13th February,2004.

Varshney,J.P. and Ram Naresh (2004). Evaluation of a homeopathic complex in the clinical management of udder diseases of riverine buffaloes. Homeopathy 93:17-20.

Varshney, J.P. (2005 a). Hepatoprotective efficacy of a homeopathic combination remedy in phenobarbital induced hepatopathy in epileptic dogs. Natn.Seminar Homeopathic Medicine Plant, Animals and Fishes, Thrissur,5-6th February, 05,pp1-5.

Varshney, J.P. (2005b). Prospects of Homeopathy in Veterinary Medicine in India.National Workshop under ASCAD on use of Alternative Systems of Medicine (Ayurvedic and Homeopathic) in Veterinary Practice, Nagpur, May 5-6, 05, pp 14-19.

Varshney, J.P. (2005c). Reversal of paroxysmal atrial tachycardia with oral administration of Digitalis 6C in dogs. International conference on "Actual points for Veterinary Homeopathy", St.Petersburg, Russia, December 20-24, 2005.

Varshney,J.P. and Ram Naresh (2005).Comparative efficacy of homeopathic andallopathic systems of medicine in the management of clinical mastitis of Indian dairy cows. Homeopathy 94:81-85.

Varshney, J.P. and Saghar, S.Soja (2005).Evaluation of hepatoprotective efficacy of a homeo-complex in dogs with hepatopathy. International Conference on "Actual points for Veterinary Homeopathy", St.Petersburg, Russia, December 20-24, 2005.

Varshney, J.P.(2006 a). Thelitis in Dairy Animals. Homeopathic Links .International Journal of Classical Homeopathy Winter 19:218 @ SonntagVerlog in MVS,Medizinverlage GmbH & Co. KG

Varshney,J.P.(2006b). Clinical Management of Canine Viral Gastroenteritis with a HomeopathicCombination Remedy. In: Research Findings. Homeopathic Bioefficacy and Management of Animal Health. Varshney, J.P. and Swaminarayan, S (eds). Sintex International Limited, Kalol, pp.115-119.

Varshney, J.P. (2006 c). Arsenic album in gastroenteritis in pups.Am.J.Homeopathic Medicine (Winter Issue) 2006 ,99(4):296-297.

Varshney, J.P. (2006 d). Clinical management of idiopathic epilepsy in dogs with homeopathic Belladonna 200C; a case series . Homeopathy 96:46-48.

Varshney, J.P.(2007a). Clinical Management of Acute Mastitis in Bitches with a Homeo-Complex. In: Research Findings. Homeopathic Bioefficacy and Management of Animal Health. Varshney, J.P. and Swaminarayan, S (eds). Sintex International Limited, Kalol, pp.55-59.

Vatshney,J.P.(2007b). Hepatoprotective Efficacy of A Homeopathic Combination Remedy in Phenobarbital Induced Hepatopathy in Epileptic Dogs). In: Research Findings. Homeopathic Bioefficacy and Management of Animal Health. Varshney, J.P. and Swaminarayan, S (eds). Sintex International Limited, Kalol, pp.25-28.

Varshney, J.P. (2007c) .Clinical Management of Haematuria with Uva ursi. In: Research Findings. Homeopathic Bioefficacy and Management of Animal Health. Varshney, J.P. and Swaminarayan, S (eds). Sintex International Limited, Kalol, pp.101-102.

Varshney, J.P.(2007d). Clinical Management of Haematuria with a Homeopathic-complex in a Spitz Dog. In: Research Findings. Homeopathic Bioefficacy and Management of

Animal Health. Varshney, J.P. and Swaminarayan, S (eds). Sintex International Limited, Kalol, pp.103-105.

Varshney, J.P. (2007e) . A preliminary trial of a homeopathic shampoo in the management of Seborrhoea in Dogs. In: Research Findings.Homeopathic Bioefficacy and Management of Animal Health. Varshney, J.P. and Swaminarayan, S (eds). Sintex International Limited, Kalol, pp 125-127.

Varshney, J.P. (2007 f). Clinical management of cystitis in dogs with Cantheris. In: Research Findings. Homeopathic Bioefficacy and Management of Animal Health. Varshney, J.P. and Swaminarayan, S (eds). Sintex International Limited, Kalol, pp 106-109..

Varshney, J.P. and Chaudhuri, S. (2007). Atrial paroxysmal tachycardia in dogs andits management with homeopathic digitalis.- Two case report. Homeopathy 96 (4) :270-272.

Varshne, J.P.,Deshmukh ,V.V.and Chaudhary,P.S. (2007). Clinical Management of common cold in a Labrador pup with Allium cepa 30C.. 15th All India Homeopathic Scientific Seminar, Rajkot, 21-23rd Dec.,2007.

Varshney, J.P. and Paliwal, O.P. (2007).Clinical Management of Squamous Metaplasia with Thuja in a Dog. In: Research Findings. Homeopathic Bioefficacy and Management of Animal Health. Varshney, J.P. and Swaminarayan, S (eds). Sintex InternationalLimited, Kalol, pp.148-149.

Varshney,J.P., Tandon, S.K. and Dudhgaonkar (2007).Anti-inflammatory Activity of a Homeo-complex in Carrageenan Induced Hindpaw Odema in Rats. In: Research Findings. Homeopathic Bioefficacy and Management of Animal Health. Varshney, J.P. and Swaminarayan, S. (eds). Sintex International Limited, Kalol, pp.29-33.

Varshney,J.P., Tandon,S.K. and Bhat, A.S. (2007).Evaluation of Anti-pyretic Efficacy of Homeopathic Drugs in Brewer's Yeast Induced Pyrexia.In: Research Findings. Homeopathic Bioefficacy and Management of Animal Health. Varshney, J.P. and Swaminarayan, S. (eds). Sintex International Limited, Kalol, pp.96-10.

Varshney,J.P., Paliwal, O.P. and Hoque, M. (2007).Use of A Homeo-complex as An Adjunct Therapy in the Management of Infectious Canine Hepatitis. In: Research Findings. Homeopathic Bioefficacy and Management of Animal Health. Varshney, J.P. and Swaminarayan, S (eds). Sintex International Limited, Kalol, pp.60-63.

Varshney,J.P.and Swaminarayan, S.(2010) . Homeopathic drugs in the managementof anaemia in animals. Brain Storming Session at CFTRI , Mysore

Varshney, J.P. and Swaminarayan,S, (2010). Clinical management of gastroenteritis with Arsenic album 30C in animals. XXII National Congress ofIndian Institute of Homeopathic Physicians, Delhi State Branch, Delhi

Varshney,J.P. (2011).An overview of Research in Homeopathic Veterinary Medicine in India. Liga 2011

Varshney, J.P.(2011).Diagnosis and Management of Atrial Paroxysmal Tachycardia in Dogs with Homeopathic Digitalis. Liga 2011

Varshney, J.P. and Swaminarayan, S. (2011) Clinical Management of Thelitis with homeopathic drugs in cows and buffaloes. Liga 2011.

Varshney, J.P. nd Swaminarayan, S.(2011). Clinical Management of Gastroenteritis with Arsenic album 30C in animals Asian Conference held at Ceylon.

Varshney, J.P. (2013). Clinical management of haematuric dogs with Cantheris 30C.Journal of Case Studies in Homeopathy.1 (2):2-6.

Varshney , J.P.(2016). Management of Osteoarthritis in dogs using a homeopathic combination remedy. Indian.J. Vet.Med. 36:148-150.

Varshney,J.P. and Swaminarayan,S. (2018). Case Study: Canine Bladder Tumour (Transitional Cell Carcinoma). 3rd International Conference on Integrative Oncology. Nashik (19-21 Jan, 2018).

Varshney, J. P. (2024 a). Management of Transitional Cell Carcinoma in dogs with Homeopathic Calcarea carbonica. (personal communication).

Varshney,J.P.(2024b).Clinical Management of Suppurative-arthritis in crossbred calf with a Homeopathic Combination Remedy after drainage (personal communication).

Varshney,J.P. (2024c).Clinical Management of aural hematoma with Arnica montana and Hamamelis virginica (personal communication).

Varshney,J.P.(2024d).Clinical Management of non-suppurative wounds in animalswith Homeopathic Calendula cream (personal communication).

Varshney,J. P.(2024 e). Clinical Management of Marked Epiphora with Euphrasia 10 % eye solution in kittens (personal communication).

Varshney,J. P. (2024 f). Orexigenic Potential of Homopathic Alfalfa Q in Turtles (personal communication).

Varshney,J. P. (2024 g). Feline icterus owing to Hepatic Lipidosis Treated with Chelidonium 30 c (personal communication).

Varshney,J. P. (2024 h). Clinical Management of Neck Trauma in a kitten with Homeopathic drugs (personal communication).

Varshney,J.P. (2024 i).Clinical Trial with Homeopathic drugs in chronic cases of Pseudomonas Otitis Media in dogs (personal communication).

Varshney,J.P. (2024 j). Clinical Management of Corneal Ulcers in dogs with Silica terra 30c and Euphrasia 10 % eye solution (personal communication).

Varshney,J.P. (2024 k). Clinical Management of Seborrhea sicca in Dogs with Sulphur 30c (personal communication)